MAKERS OF MODERN BIOMEDICINE: A REGISTER

Compiled by C Overy, A Wilkinson, and E M Tansey

Volume 63   2017

First published by Queen Mary University of London, 2017

The History of Modern Biomedicine Research Group is funded by the Wellcome Trust, which is a registered charity, no. 210183.

ISBN 978 1 91019 5307

All volumes are freely available online at www.histmodbiomed.org

Please cite as: Overy C, Wilkinson A, Tansey E M. (comps) (2017) *Makers of Modern Biomedicine: A Register.* Wellcome Witnesses to Contemporary Medicine, vol. 63. London: Queen Mary University of London.

CONTENTS

INTRODUCTION

In 1997 we published the proceedings of our first four Witness Seminars in modern medicine, funded by the Wellcome Trust. Somewhat optimistically, we called this 'volume 1', hoping that we might get funding and support to develop the series at least into double figures. After twenty years of generous funding, we have now published 62 volumes, containing the proceedings of 70 or so seminars, all of which are made freely available on the web.

The themes represented here were selected by a Programme Committee (until 2010) or were related to a Strategic Award from the Wellcome Trust (from 2010 until 2017). Topics cover the whole range of modern biomedicine: from clinical genetics to medical- and bio-technology; ethics to rural practice; pure lab research to clinical care; narrative medicine to neuroscience. Our meetings have attracted more than 1200 individuals who have contributed their recollections and comments, agreements and disagreements; several of them having contributed in multiple ways: attending or chairing a number of meetings, writing introductions to the published proceedings, providing commentaries and appendices.

Additionally, we have conducted further interviews with more than 65 people, either on audio or video, and usually both. Most, but not all, of these interviewees, have been previous participants at one or more Witness Seminars, and we have used an in-depth interview to enlarge upon experiences and views expressed in those seminars, to develop broader contexts, and to explore individual experiences in more detail. As with the Witness Seminars, all these interviews have been transcribed and edited, and made freely available online; and a small selection has been further edited and published as *Voices of Modern Biomedicine.*

One thing that emerges clearly from this work is that there is no such thing as 'an ordinary life', and we are enormously grateful to the many men and women who have trusted us with their memories, and contributed to one or both of our recording projects.

We now conclude the published Witness Seminar series with a register of the many people who have taken part in our meetings. Firstly, there is an alphabetical list of all participants, with a reference to the meeting(s) to which they contributed or to their individual interview. Secondly, we provide thumbnail portraits usually taken in the course of our Seminars or interviews. This list is not complete as not all participants were photographed, or provided copyright permission to use their images. Most portraits are available in colour at http://www.histmodbiomed.org/witsem/vol63.

Tilli Tansey
School of History,
Queen Mary University of London

Short title	Full title	Vol No.
Medical Ethics	Medical ethics education in Britain, 1963–1993	31
Ethics of Genetics.	Medical genetics: development of ethical dimensions in clinical practice and research	57
Migraine	Migraine: diagnosis, treatment and understanding c.1960–2010	49
Monoclonal Antibodies	Technology transfer in Britain: the case of monoclonal antibodies	1
MRSA	Superbugs and superdrugs: a history of MRSA	32
Muscular Dystrophy	The therapeutic implications of muscular dystrophy genomics	62
Narrative Medicine	The development of narrative practices in medicine c.1960–c.2000	52
NATSAL	History of the National Survey of Sexual Attitudes and Lifestyles	41
Neonatal Intensive Care	Neonatal intensive care	9
NIMR	Technology, techniques, and technicians at the National Institute for Medical Research (NIMR) c.1960–c.2000	59
NMR and MRI	Making the human body transparent: The impact of NMR and MRI	2
Pain	Innovation in pain management	21
Palliative Medicine	Palliative medicine in the UK c.1970–2010	45
Peptic Ulcer	Peptic ulcer: Rise and fall	14
Platelets	The recent history of platelets in thrombosis and other disorders	23
Platinum Salts	The discovery, use and impact of platinum salts as chemotherapy agents for cancer	30
Population-based Research	Population-based research in south Wales: The MRC Pneumoconiosis Research Unit and the MRC Epidemiology Unit	13

Dr Catherine Belling
(b. 1965), medical humanities scholar:
Narrative Medicine.

Dr Barry Benster
(b. 1937), obstetrician and
gynaecologist:
Rhesus Factor.

Dame Valerie Beral
(b. 1946), epidemiologist:
Cervical Cancer.

Professor Virginia Berridge
(b. 1946), medical historian:
*Cannabis, Endogenous Opiates, NATSAL,
Public Health, Tobacco Control.*

Dr Caroline Berry
(b. 1937), clinical geneticist:
Clinical Genetics.

Professor Sir Colin Berry
(b. 1937), pathologist:
Environmental Toxicology.

Dr Douglas Bettcher
(b. 1956), public health specialist:
Tobacco Control.

Professor John Betteridge
(b. 1948), endocrinologist:
Cholesterol.

Professor Sanjoy Bhattacharya
(b. 1968), medical historian:
Tobacco Control.

Dr Ethel Bidwell
(1919–2003), research scientist in
blood coagulation:
Haemophilia.

Mr Brian Biles
(1926–2016) electron microscopist:
Individual Interview.

Professor Julian Bion
(b. 1952), intensive care specialist:
Intensive Care.

Mr Simon Birkett
(b. 1959), campaigner:
Air Pollution.

Miss Karen Birmingham
(b. 1955), Secretary of Ethics and Law
Committee:
ALSPAC.

Professor Timothy Bishop
(b. 1953), cancer geneticist:
Gene Mapping, Clinical Cancer Genetics.

Sir Douglas Black
(1913–2002), physician, civil servant:
Clinical Research.

Professor Sir James Black
(1924–2010), pharmacologist, Nobel
Laureate (1988):
Clinical Pharmacology 1, Peptic Ulcer.

Professor Nick Black
(b. 1951), health services researcher:
Public Health.

Dr Tom Blackburn
(b. 1949), industrial pharmacologist:
5-HT, Migraine, Individual Interview.

Professor Roland Blackwell
(b. 1943), medical physicist:
*Medical Physics, Neonatal Intensive
Care.*

Professor Christopher Blagg
(b. 1931), nephrologist and medical
director:
Dialysis.

Miss Anthea Blake
(b. 1942), neonatal nurse:
Neonatal Intensive Care.

Professor David Blane
(b. 1945), physician and social scientist:
Public Health.

Dr Joseph N Blau
(1928–2010), neurologist:
Medical Physics, Peptic Ulcer.

Professor Martin Bobrow
(b. 1938), geneticist:
*Clinical Genetics, Clinical Molecular
Genetics.*

Professor Sir Walter Bodmer
(b. 1936), geneticist:
Clinical Cancer Genetics, Gene Mapping.

Professor Sir Michael Bond
(b. 1936), consultant psychiatrist:
Pain.

Dr Tim Boon
(b. 1960), museum curator:
Common Cold Unit.

Sir Christopher Booth
(1924–2012), gastroenterologist,
research director and medical
historian:
*Africa, Asthma, Applied Psychology,
Autoimmunity, Cholesterol, Clinical
Research, Common Cold Unit,
Corticosteroids, Cystic Fibrosis, Dialysis,
Environmental Toxicology, General
Practice, Genetic Testing, Haemophilia,
Heart Transplant, Hip Replacement,
Intestinal Absorption, Leukaemia,
Maternal Care, Medical Ethics, Medical
Physics, Monoclonal Antibodies,
Neonatal Intensive Care, NMR and
MRI, Peptic Ulcer, Platelets, Population-
based Research, Post Penicillin,
Psychiatric Drugs, Safety of Drugs, TB
Chemotherapy.*

Professor Gustav Born
(b. 1921), pharmacologist:
Cholesterol, Platelets.

Dr Malcolm Bottomley
(b. 1933), GP:
Sports Medicine.

Dr Frank Boulton
(b. 1941), haematologist:
Rhesus Factor.

Mrs Ruth Bowles
(b. 1960), ALSPAC parent, research
nurse and member of ALSPAC Law
and Ethics Committee:
ALSPAC.

Professor Kenneth Boyd
(b. 1939), medical ethicist:
Medical Ethics.

Dr Richard Boyd
(b. 1945), physiologist:
Cystic Fibrosis, Intestinal Absorption.

Professor Sir Robert Boyd
(b. 1938), paediatrician:
Neonatal Intensive Care.

Professor David Bradley
(b. 1937), professor of tropical
medicine:
Africa.

Professor Ronald Bradley
(b. 1929), intensive therapy medicine
specialist:
Intensive Care.

Miss Mary Brancker
(1914–2010), President of the British
Veterinary Association – 1967/8 foot
and mouth disease outbreak:
Foot and Mouth.

Dr Margaret Branthwaite
(b. 1935), consultant anaesthetist:
Intensive Care.

Professor Carol Brayne
(b. 1957), professor of public health
and epidemiologist:
Brain Banks.

Sir Alasdair Breckenridge
(b. 1937), pharmacologist:
Clinical Pharmacology 2.

Professor Leslie Brent
(b. 1925), immunologist:
Autoimmunity, Foot and Mouth.

Dr Alistair Brewis
(1937–2014), respiratory physician:
Asthma.

Dr Alan Broadhurst
(b. 1926), consultant psychiatrist:
Psychiatric Drugs.

Dr Penelope Brock
(b. 1954), consultant paediatric
oncologist:
Platinum Salts.

Dr Peter Brocklehurst
(b. 1962), obstetrician and
gynaecologist/epidemiologist:
Corticosteroids.

Professor Jens Brockmeier
(b. 1951), psychology and linguistics
scholar:
Narrative Medicine.

Professor J Ramsey Bronk
(1929–2007), professor of
biochemistry:
Intestinal Absorption.

Dr Ivan Brown
(1927–2014), psychologist:
Applied Psychology.

Professor Morris Brown
(b. 1951), pharmacologist:
Clinical Pharmacology 1.

Mr Thomas Brown
(b. 1933), engineer:
Ultrasound.

Dr Doreen Browne
(b. 1934), consultant anaesthetist:
Intensive Care.

Professor Richard Bruckdorfer
(b. 1942), biochemist:
Cholesterol.

Dr Linda Bryder
(b. 1956), medical historian:
TB Chemotherapy.

Mrs Phyll Buchanan
(b. 1957), founder member and
trustee of the National Childcare
Trust. Breastfeeding Network:
Breastfeeding.

Dr Robert Bud
(b. 1952), museum curator, medical
historian:
*Monoclonal Antibodies, MRSA, Post
Penicillin.*

Professor Petar Bulat
(b. 1961), occupational toxicologist:
Rural Medicine.

Dr Michael Bull
(1926–2013), hospital practitioner in
obstetrics:
Maternal Care.

Professor Arthur Buller
(b. 1923), chief scientist DHSS:
Clinical Research.

Professor John Bunker
(1920–2012), anaesthetist:
Heart Transplant.

Dr Geoff Bunn
(b. 1968), historian:
Applied Psychology.

Professor Terence Burlin
(b. 1931), physicist:
Medical Physics.

Professor Sir John Burn
(b. 1952), clinical geneticist:
*Clinical Cancer Genetics, Clinical
Genetics.*

Dr Ian Burney
(b. 1962), medical historian:
Sports Medicine.

Mr J E (Bob) Burns
(b. 1928), medical physicist:
Medical Physics.

Professor Geoffrey Burnstock
(b. 1929), neuroscientist:
Individual Interview.

Dr Michael Burr
(b. 1937), epidemiologist:
Population-based Research.

Professor Kate Bushby
(b. 1962), neuromuscular geneticist:
Muscular Dystrophy.

Professor Graeme Bydder
(b. 1944), radiologist:
NMR and MRI.

Mr Timothy Byrne
(b. 1979), waste manager:
Waste.

Dr Eric Bywaters
(1910–2003), rheumatologist:
Clinical Research.

Fr Brendan Callaghan
(b. 1948), medical ethicist:
Medical Ethics.

Dr Sheila Callender
(1914–2004), haematologist:
Intestinal Absorption.

Sir Kenneth Calman
(b. 1941), oncologist/Chief Medical
Officer:
*Medical Ethics, Palliative Medicine,
Platinum Salts.*

Professor Hilary Calvert
(b. 1947), medical oncologist:
Platinum Salts.

Professor Dugald Cameron
(b. 1939), industrial designer:
Ultrasound, Individual Interview.

Professor Stewart Cameron
(b. 1934), nephrologist:
Dialysis.

Professor Alastair Campbell
(b. 1938), bioethicist:
Medical Ethics.

Dr Ian Campbell
(b. 1944), chest physician:
TB Chemotherapy.

Professor Peter Campbell
(1921–2005), biochemical
immunologist:
Autoimmunity.

Professor Stuart Campbell
(b. 1936), obstetrician and
gynaecologist:
Ultrasound.

Professor Saveria Campo
(b. 1947), viral oncologist:
Cervical Cancer.

Dr David Carnegie
(b. 1917), anaesthetist:
Heart Transplant.

Professor Richard Carter
(b. 1934), histopathologist:
Environmental Toxicology.

Dr Tim Carter
(b. 1944), occupational health
specialist:
Public Health.

Professor Ann Cartwright
(b. 1925), statistician and socio–
medical researcher:
General Practice.

Professor Mark Casewell
(1940–2011), medical microbiologist:
MRSA.

Dr Angela Cassidy
(b. 1975), historian of science:
Bovine TB.

Professor Daniel Catovsky
(b. 1937), consultant haematologist:
Leukaemia.

Dr William Cattell
(b. 1928), nephrologist:
Dialysis.

Professor Mark Caulfield
(b. 1960), pharmacologist:
Clinical Pharmacology 1.

Dr Sandy Cavenagh
(1929–2014), GP obstetrician:
Maternal Care.

Mr Roger Celestin
(b. 1925), surgeon:
Peptic Ulcer.

Professor Sir Iain Chalmers
(b. 1943), Director – UK Cochrane
Centre (1992–2002) / National
Perinatal Epidemiology Unit
(1978–1992):
*Clinical Pharmacology 1, Clinical
Pharmacology 2, Corticosteroids,
Maternal Care, Public Health, TB
Chemotherapy.*

Professor Geoffrey Chamberlain
(1930–2014), obstetrician and
gynaecologist:
Maternal Care.

Professor Jocelyn Chamberlain
(b. 1932), epidemiologist:
Cervical Cancer.

Professor Donald Chambers
(b. 1937), biochemist:
Platelets.

Mr Geof Chambers
(b. 1955), mechanical engineer:
NIMR.

Dr Donna Chaproniere
(b. 1929), virologist:
Common Cold Unit.

Lady Jill Charnley
(d. 2016), Widow of Sir John Charnley
(1911–1982), orthopaedic surgeon,
pioneer of hip replacement surgery:
Hip Replacement.

Mr Tristram Charnley
(b. 1959), Son of Sir John Charnley
(1911–1982), orthopaedic surgeon,
pioneer of hip replacement surgery:
Hip Replacement.

Professor Rita Charon
(b. 1949), practitioner of general
internal medicine and narrative
medicine:
Narrative Medicine.

Professor Bruce Chater
(b. 1956), rural physician:
Rural Medicine.

Dr Bilwanath Chattopadhyay
(b. 1939), medical microbiologist:
MRSA.

Dr Ian Lister Cheese
(b. 1936), senior civil servant in the
(UK) Department of Health:
*ALSPAC, Clinical Genetics, Clinical
Molecular Genetics.*

Professor Yuti Chernajovsky
(b. 1954), cancer biologist:
TNF.

Dr Daphne Christie, medical
historian:
Breastfeeding, Medical Ethics.

Dr Kenneth Citron
(b. 1925), respiratory physician,
Chairman of British Thoracic Society's
Tuberculosis Clinical Trials Committee:
TB Chemotherapy.

Professor David Clark
(b. 1953), medical sociologist:
Pain, Palliative Medicine.

Dr John Clark, medical historian:
Environmental Toxicology.

Mr Michael Clark
(b. 1943), wildlife field worker and
artist:
Bovine TB.

Professor Tim Clark
(b. 1935), professor of pulmonary
medicine:
Asthma.

Dr Aileen Clarke
(b. 1955), public health specialist:
Public Health.

Professor Angus Clarke
(b. 1954), clinical geneticist:
Clinical Genetics, Ethics of Genetics.

Professor David Clarke
(b. 1936), pharmacologist:
5-HT.

Professor John Clifton
(b. 1930), medical physicist:
Medical Physics.

Professor Forrester Cockburn
(b. 1934), paediatrician:
Breastfeeding.

Ms Marjory Cockburn
(b. 1927), hospice nurse:
Palliative Medicine.

Dr Chris Coggins
(b. 1947–2017), waste management
academic:
Waste, Individual Interview.

Dr Nelson Coghill
(1912–2002), gastroenterologist:
Peptic Ulcer.

Professor Jon Cohen
physician and infectious diseases
expert:
TNF

Dr Martin Cole
(b. 1933), microbiologist:
Post Penicillin.

Professor Dulcie Coleman
(b. 1932), consultant cytopathologist:
Cervical Cancer.

Professor Joe Collier
(b. 1942), clinical pharmacologist,
President of the International Society
of Drug Bulletins:
Clinical Pharmacology 2.

Professor Leslie Collier
(1921–2011), virologist:
Clinical Research.

Mr Eric Collins
(b. 1936), pharmaceutical sales
engineer:
Dialysis.

Mr Neil Collishaw
(b. 1946), lead tobacco control expert
for WHO's 'Tobacco or Health'
programme:
Tobacco Control.

Dr Brian Colvin
(b. 1946), consultant haematologist:
Haemophilia.

Dr Brian Commins
(b. 1930), research chemist:
Air Pollution.

Dr Gordon Cook
(b. 1932), tropical disease physician:
Africa, Clinical Research.

Professor Richard Cooke
(b. 1947), professor of neonatal
medicine:
Neonatal Intensive Care.

Professor Robin Coombs
(1921–2006), immunologist:
Autoimmunity, Rhesus Factor.

Mr Jeff Cooper
(b. 1949), consultant in environmental
management:
Waste, Individual Interview.

Dr Peter Corcoran
(b. 1939), physicist:
Environmental Toxicology.

Dr Beryl Corner
(1910–2007), paediatrician:
Neonatal Intensive Care, Rhesus Factor.

Professor Ian Couper
(b. 1961), professor of rural health:
Rural Medicine.

Dr Angela Coutts
pharmacologist:
Endogenous Opiates.

Professor Phillip Cowen
(b. 1951), psychopharmacologist:
5-HT, SAD.

Professor Helen Cox
(b. 1957), pharmacologist:
5-HT.

Dr Jim Cox
(1931–2001), director of research and
development in the pharmaceutical
industry:
Asthma.

Dr Jim Cox
(b. 1950), rural GP:
Rural Medicine.

Mr Michael Cox
(b. 1929), volunteer at the MRC
Common Cold Unit:
Common Cold Unit.

Professor Tony Coxon
(1938–2012), Co–director of the
Institute for Behavioural Research on
AIDS (Wales):
NATSAL.

Professor Ian Craig
(b. 1943), molecular geneticist:
Gene Mapping.

Mr Harry Craven
(1928–2007), industrial engineer:
Hip Replacement.

Dr Lionel Crawford
(b. 1932), molecular virologist:
Cervical Cancer.

Dr Gerard Crean
(1927–2005), consultant physician:
Peptic Ulcer.

Professor Arthur Crisp
(1930–2006), psychiatrist:
Psychiatric Drugs.

Professor Sir John Crofton
(1912–2009), professor of respiratory
diseases and tuberculosis:
Post Penicillin, TB Chemotherapy.

Dr Donald Crombie
(1922–2000), GP:
General Practice.

Professor Ilana Crome
(b. 1951), psychiatrist:
SAD.

Mrs Mary Cronk
(b. 1932), midwife:
Maternal Care.

Dr Patricia Crowley
(b. 1951), consultant obstetrician and
gynaecologist:
Corticosteroids.

Dr June Crown
(b. 1938), public health specialist:
Public Health.

Professor Derek Crowther
(b. 1937), oncologist:
Leukaemia.

Professor Heather Cubie
(b. 1946), bacteriologist:
Cervical Cancer.

Mr Rob Cunningham
(b. 1964), lawyer and policy adviser:
Tobacco Control.

Professor Gerald Curzon
(b. 1928), neurochemist:
5-HT, Psychiatric Drugs.

Professor Alan Cuthbert
(1932–2016), pharmacologist:
Cystic Fibrosis.

Professor Jack Cuzick
(b. 1948), epidemiologist:
Cervical Cancer.

Dr Vera Luiza da Costa e Silva
(b. 1952), public health specialist:
Tobacco Control.

Dr Ann Dally
(1926–2007), psychiatrist, medical
historian:
Maternal Care.

Dr Stephanie Dancer
(b. 1959), medical microbiologist:
MRSA.

Dr Booth Danesh
(b. 1942), consultant gastroenterologist:
Peptic Ulcer.

Professor Janet Darbyshire
(b. 1947), epidemiologist:
TB Chemotherapy.

Ms Clare Darrah
(b. 1958), clinical research manager:
Hip Replacement.

Professor Naomi Datta
(1922–2008), microbial geneticist:
Post Penicillin.

Professor George Davey Smith
(b. 1959), clinical epidemiologist:
ALSPAC, Cholesterol, Population-based Research.

Dr Hamish Davidson
(b. 1926), consultant physician:
Africa.

Professor David Davies
(1923–2002), clinical pharmacologist:
Safety of Drugs.

Professor Donald Davies
(b. 1940), biochemical pharmacologist:
Clinical Pharmacology 1, Clinical Pharmacology 2.

Mr Gareth Davies
(b. 1935), veterinary epidemiologist:
Bovine TB, Foot and Mouth.

Professor John Elfed Davies
(b. 1941), consultant physician:
Sports Medicine.

Dr Pamela Davies
(1924–2009), consultant paediatrician:
Neonatal Intensive Care.

Dr Peter Davies
(b. 1949), chest physician:
TB Chemotherapy.

Professor John Davis
(b. 1923), paediatrician:
Neonatal Intensive Care.

Dr Clare Davison
(b. 1934), clinical geneticist:
Clinical Genetics.

Professor Tony Dayan
(b. 1935), toxicologist:
Environmental Toxicology.

Mrs Rosemary de Rossi
(b. 1931), head lab technician in Immunology:
NIMR.

Dr Mahes de Silva
(b. 1943), immunohaematologist:
Rhesus Factor.

Mr Graham Deane
(b. 1939), orthopaedic surgeon:
Hip Replacement.

Professor Joy Delhanty
(b. 1937), clinical cytogeneticist:
Clinical Genetics, Genetic Testing.

Professor Sergio Della Sala
(b. 1955), neuropsychologist/neurologist:
Applied Psychology.

Professor David Delpy
(b. 1948), medical physicist:
Neonatal Intensive Care, NMR and MRI.

Dr Philip Dendy
(b. 1938), radiobiologist:
Medical Physics.

Mr Barry Dennis
(b. 1946), waste management director:
Waste, Individual Interview.

Dr Nick Dennis
(b. 1944), clinical geneticist:
Clinical Genetics, Ethics of Genetics.

Dr Christopher Derrett
(b. 1947), retired GP:
Air Pollution, Individual Interview.

Professor Richard Derwent
(b. 1947), physical chemist:
Air Pollution.

Dr Hewan Dewar
(1913–2012), cardiologist:
Platelets.

Dr Vincenzo Di Marzo
(b. 1960), pharmacologist:
Cannabis.

Professor Donna Dickenson
(b. 1946), medical ethicist:
Medical Ethics.

Professor John Dickinson
(1927–2015), pharmacologist,
physician:
Clinical Research, Platelets.

Professor George Dickson
(b. 1953), molecular cell biologist:
Muscular Dystrophy.

Dr Angela Dike
(b. 1936), haematologist and
pathologist:
Haemophilia.

Mr Ross Dike
(b. 1932), laboratory research worker:
Haemophilia.

Professor Nigel Dimmock
(b. 1940), virologist:
Common Cold Unit.

Dr Bernard Dixon
(b. 1938), science journalist:
MRSA.

Professor Thomas Dixon
(b. 1973), historian:
SAD.

Professor Mary Dobson
(b. 1954), medical historian:
Africa.

Professor Graham Dockray
(b. 1946), gastric physiologist:
Peptic Ulcer.

Mrs Mary Dodd
(b. 1944), consultant physiotherapist:
Cystic Fibrosis.

Ms Rosie Dodds
nutritionist:
Breastfeeding.

Professor John Dodge
(b. 1933), paediatrician:
Cystic Fibrosis.

Dr Helen Dodsworth
(b. 1938), consultant physician and
haematologist:
Haemophilia.

Professor Sir Richard Doll
(1912–2005), statistician and
epidemiologist:
*Peptic Ulcer, Platelets, Population-based
Research.*

Mrs Alix Donald
(1918–2008), widow of Professor
Ian Donald (1910–1987), obstetrician:
Ultrasound.

Professor Deborah Doniach
(1912–2004), clinical immunologist:
Autoimmunity.

Professor Israel Doniach
(1911–2001), immunologist and
pathologist:
Autoimmunity.

Professor Dian Donnai
(b. 1945), medical geneticist:
Clinical Genetics.

Dr Jean Donnison
(1925–2017), social policy
administrator:
Maternal Care.

Professor Tony Dornhorst
(1915–2003), professor of medicine:
Clinical Research.

Dr James Douglas
(b. 1951), rural GP:
Rural Medicine.

Professor Stuart Douglas
(1921–1998), physician:
Haemophilia.

Dr Colin Dourish
(b. 1955), psychopharmacologist:
5-HT.

Professor Hermon Dowling
(b. 1934), gastroenterologist:
Intestinal Absorption.

Dr Peter Down
(b. 1939), gastroenterologist:
Peptic Ulcer.

Professor Duncan Dowson
(b. 1928), mechanical engineer:
Hip Replacement.

Dr Peter Doyle
(1921–2004), industrial pharmaceutical
chemist:
Post Penicillin.

Dr Christopher Draper
(1921–2006), consultant in tropical
hygiene:
Africa.

Professor James Drife
(b. 1947), obstetrician and
gynaecologist:
Maternal Care.

Professor Sir Michael Drury
(1926–2014), GP:
General Practice.

Dr Lilly Dubowitz
(1930–2016), paediatrician:
Neonatal Intensive Care.

Professor Victor Dubowitz
(b. 1931), paediatrician:
*Neonatal Intensive Care, Muscular
Dystrophy, Individual Interview.*

Dr Georgia Duckworth
(b. 1954), veterinary microbiologist:
MRSA.

Professor Brian Duerden
(b. 1948), microbiologist:
MRSA.

Dr Tony Duggan
(1920–2004), tropical medicine
expert:
Africa.

Mr David C Duncan
(b. 1926), psychologist:
Applied Psychology.

Dr Ian Duncan
(b. 1943), gynaecological oncologist:
Cervical Cancer.

Dr Sheila Duncan
(b. 1931), obstetrician/gynaecologist:
Maternal Care, Rhesus Factor.

Mrs Fran Duncan-Skingle
(b. 1939), cystic fibrosis clinical nurse
specialist:
Cystic Fibrosis.

Professor Peter Dunn
(b. 1929), paediatrician:
Maternal Care, Neonatal Intensive Care.

Dame Karen Dunnell
(b. 1946), statistician:
NATSAL.

Mr Mike Durham
(b. 1952), journalist:
NATSAL.

Professor Paul Durrington
(b. 1947), researcher in lipoprotein
metabolism:
Cholesterol.

Professor Robert Duthie
(1925–2005), orthopaedic surgeon:
Haemophilia.

Miss Caroline Dux
(b. 1955), neonatal nurse:
Neonatal Intensive Care.

Mrs Jill Dye
(b. 1949), lactation consultant:
Breastfeeding.

Professor Fiona Dykes
(b. 1960), nutrition researcher:
Breastfeeding.

Mrs Ann Eady
(b. 1944), dialysis nurse:
Dialysis.

Professor Robin Eady
(b. 1940), dermatologist and dialysis
patient:
Dialysis.

Ms Jennifer Eastwood
(b. 1952), founder of SADA:
SAD.

Dr Friedericke Eben
(b. 1956), obstetrician:
Maternal Care.

Dr Demetrios Economides
(b. 1956), obstetrician:
Ultrasound.

Professor Griffith Edwards
(1928–2012), drugs adviser:
Cannabis.

Professor John Edwards
(1928–2007), geneticist:
Genetic Testing.

Mrs Sheila Edwards
(b. 1947), daughter of J N 'Ginger'
Wilson, orthopaedic surgeon:
Hip Replacement.

Dr Andrew Elder
(b. 1945), GP, trainer, and educator:
Narrative Medicine.

Dr Rob Elles
(b. 1951), molecular geneticist:
Clinical Molecular Genetics.

Miss Freda Ellis
(b. 1931), ward sister:
Dialysis.

Dr Niki Ellis
sociologist:
Pain.

Dr Giles Elrington
(b. 1956), consultant neurologist:
Migraine.

Mr Reg Elson
(b. 1930), orthopaedic surgeon:
Hip Replacement.

Professor Peter Elwood
(b. 1930), Director of the MRC
Epidemiological Research Unit in
South Wales:
*Platelets, Population-based Research,
Individual Interview.*

Professor Alan Emery
(b. 1928), medical geneticist:
Clinical Genetics.

Mr Steve Eminton
environmental journalist:
Waste.

Professor Michael Emmerson
(1937–2008), medical microbiologist:
MRSA.

Professor Alan Emond
(b. 1953), paediatrician:
ALSPAC.

Ms Hilary English
breastfeeding counsellor:
Breastfeeding.

Sir Terence English
(b. 1932), transplant surgeon:
Heart Transplant.

Mr Bob Erens
(b. 1953), director of social science
research programmes:
NATSAL.

Professor Margaret Esiri
(b. 1941), neuropathologist:
Brain Banks.

Dr David Evans
(b. 1930), paediatrician:
Haemophilia.

Professor Gareth Evans
(b. 1959), medical geneticist:
Clinical Cancer Genetics.

Mrs Jane Evans
(b. 1953), midwife:
Maternal Care.

Professor Douglas Eveleigh
(b. 1933), microbiologist:
Post Penicillin.

Professor Denys Fairweather
(b. 1927), obstetrician and
gynaecologist:
Neonatal Intensive Care.

Professor Peter Farmer
(b. 1947), toxicologist:
Environmental Toxicology.

Dr Philip Farrell
(b. 1943), paediatric pathologist,
epidemiologist:
Cystic Fibrosis.

Professor Bobbie Farsides
medical ethicist:
Ethics of Genetics.

Dr Alex Faulkner
(b. 1952), sociologist of medical
technology:
Hip Replacement.

Dr Joan Faulkner
(1914–2001), Senior Principal Medical
Officer, MRC:
Population-based Research.

Professor Christina Faull
(b. 1961), palliative care consultant:
Pain, Palliative Medicine.

Professor Sir Marc Feldmann
(b. 1944), immunologist:
TNF.

Mr John Ferguson
(b. 1927), waste management engineer:
Waste, Individual Interview.

Professor Malcolm Ferguson-Smith
(b. 1931), molecular geneticist:
Clinical Molecular Genetics, Gene Mapping, Genetic Testing, Individual Interview.

Professor Robin Ferner
(b. 1949), pharmacologist:
Clinical Pharmacology 1.

Dr Freda Festenstein
(b. 1927), chest physician:
TB Chemotherapy.

Mrs Julia Field
(b. 1935), principal investigator on NATSAL:
NATSAL.

Baroness Ilora Finlay
(b. 1949), palliative care specialist:
Palliative Medicine.

Professor Ronald Finn
(1930–2004), haematologist:
Rhesus Factor.

Professor David Finney
(b. 1917), statistician:
Safety of Drugs.

Dr Norman Finter
(1924–2012), virologist:
Common Cold Unit.

Ms Chloe Fisher
(b. 1932), midwife:
Breastfeeding, Maternal Care.

Dr Robert Flanagan
(b. 1948), toxicologist:
Environmental Toxicology.

Professor Alan Fleming
(b. 1931), tropical haematologist:
Africa.

Mr John Fleming
(b. 1934), medical electronics engineer:
Ultrasound.

Dr Peter Fletcher
(b. 1930), chemical pathologist:
Clinical Pharmacology 2.

Dr Tom Flewett
(1922–2006), virologist:
Common Cold Unit.

Mrs Caroline Flint
(b. 1941), midwife and former President of the Royal College of Midwives:
Maternal Care.

Professor Rod Flower
(b. 1945), pharmacologist:
5-HT, Clinical Pharmacology 1, Clinical Pharmacology 2, Platelets, Individual Interview.

Professor Sir Brian Follett
(b. 1939), endocrinologist and chronobiologist:
SAD.

Dr Gillian Ford
(b. 1934), deputy chief medical officer and medical director:
Palliative Medicine.

Sir Patrick Forrest
(b. 1923), surgeon:
Peptic Ulcer.

Dr Arthur Fowle
(b. 1929), clinical pharmacologist:
Clinical Pharmacology 1, Clinical Pharmacology 2.

Professor Jack Fowler
(b. 1925–2016), medical physicist:
Medical Physics.

Professor Renée Fox
(b. 1928), social scientist:
Heart Transplant.

Mrs Gaye Fox
widow of Wallace Fox, TB Physician:
TB Chemotherapy.

Dr Katherine Foxhall
(b. 1981), medical historian:
Migraine.

Professor Richard Frackowiak
(b. 1950), neuroscientist:
Individual Interview.

Professor Paul Francis
(b. 1958), neurochemist and Director
of Brains for Dementia Research:
Brain Banks.

Professor Arthur Frank
(b. 1946), medical sociologist:
Narrative Medicine.

Dr Bill Frankland
(b. 1912), consultant allergist:
Asthma.

Professor Ian Franklin
(b. 1949), haematologist:
Rhesus Factor.

Professor George Fraser
(b. 1932), geneticist:
*Clinical Cancer Genetics, Clinical
Genetics.*

Mrs Margaret Fraser Roberts
(b. 1927), epidemiologist:
Clinical Genetics.

Professor Paul Freeling
(1928–2002), GP:
General Practice.

Professor Michael Freeman
(b. 1931), orthopaedic surgeon:
Hip Replacement.

Professor Gary French
(b. 1945), microbiologist:
MRSA.

Dr Jeff French
(b. 1955), marketing and
communications director:
Public Health.

Dr Kathy French
(b. 1948), sexual health adviser:
NATSAL.

Professor Uta Frith
(b. 1941), psychologist:
Individual Interview.

Dr Alan Fryer
(b. 1954), paediatrician and clinical
geneticist:
Ethics of Genetics.

Mrs Iris Fudge
(b. 1927), nurse:
Medical Ethics.

Professor Bill Fulford
(b. 1942), philosopher and psychiatrist:
Medical Ethics.

Professor John Gabbay
(b. 1949), public health specialist:
Corticosteroids.

Professor David Gadian
(b. 1950), biophysicist:
NMR and MRI.

Mrs Jean Gaffin
(b. 1936), Chief Executive of National Council for Hospice and Palliative Care Services:
Palliative Medicine.

Ms Janet Gahegan
(b. 1939), Macmillan nurse:
Palliative Medicine.

Dr Michael Gait
molecular biologist:
Muscular Dystrophy.

Dr Paresh Gajjar
(b. 1945), palliative care specialist:
Palliative Medicine.

Professor Charles Galasko
(b. 1939), consultant orthopaedic surgeon:
Sports Medicine.

Professor John Galloway
(b. 1942), medical administrator:
Cannabis, Dialysis, Monoclonal Antibodies, NMR and MRI.

Professor David Galton
(1922–2006), physician, Secretary of the MRC Working Party on Leukaemia:
Leukaemia.

Professor David Galton
(b. 1937), clinical biochemist:
Cholesterol, Genetic Testing.

Professor Harold Gamsu
(1931–2004), neonatologist:
Corticosteroids, Neonatal Intensive Care.

Professor Michael Gardner
(b. 1946), professor of physiological biochemistry:
Intestinal Absorption.

Dr Tony Garland
(b. 1938), veterinary vaccinologist:
Foot and Mouth.

Mrs Diana Garratt
(b. 1960), childhood dialysis patient:
Dialysis.

Mr Hans Gassert
(b. 1944), businessman and founder of Diagnostic Sonar Limited:
Ultrasound.

Professor Duncan Geddes
(b. 1942), respiratory physician:
Cystic Fibrosis.

Professor Stanley Gelbier
(b. 1935), dentist, historian of dentistry:
Medical Ethics, Public Health.

Professor Michael Gelder
(b. 1929), psychiatrist:
Psychiatric Drugs.

Professor Curtis Gemmell
(b. 1941), bacteriologist:
MRSA.

Professor Sir Charles George
(b. 1941), pharmacologist:
Clinical Pharmacology 1, Clinical Pharmacology 2.

Professor Rob George
(b. 1953), palliative care specialist:
Palliative Medicine.

Sir Roger Gibbs
(b. 1934), Chairman of the Wellcome Trust's Board of Governors (1989–1999):
NATSAL.

Dr Tony Gilbertson
(b. 1932), consultant anaesthetist/
Director of intensive therapy units:
Intensive Care.

Dr Edward Gill
(b. 1931), pharmacologist:
Cannabis.

Professor Herbert Gilles
(1921–2015), tropical medicine
expert:
Africa.

Dr Michael Gillies
(1920–1999), medical entomologist:
Africa.

Professor Raanan Gillon
(b. 1941), medical ethicist:
Medical Ethics.

Professor Sir Ian Gilmore
(b. 1947), physician:
Intensive Care.

Dr Alan Gilston
(1928–2005), consultant anaesthetist:
Heart Transplant.

Dr David Girling
(b. 1937), chest physician:
TB Chemotherapy.

Dr Dino Giussani
(b. 1967), foetal medicine researcher:
Corticosteroids.

Dr Toni Gladding
waste management academic:
Waste.

Professor Anna Glasier
(b. 1950), professor of sexual health:
Breastfeeding.

Professor Alan Glynn
(1923–2014), bacteriologist:
*Clinical Research, Foot and Mouth,
MRSA, Post Penicillin, Public Health, TB
Chemotherapy.*

Professor Simon Godfrey
(b. 1939), paediatric respiratory
physician:
Asthma.

Professor Jean Golding
(b. 1939), Director of ALSPAC:
ALSPAC.

Professor John Goldman
(1938–2013), leukaemia specialist:
Leukaemia.

Dr John Goldsmith
(b. 1924), nephrologist:
Dialysis.

Professor Alison Goodall
(b. 1949), biochemical pathologist:
Platelets.

Dr Mary Goodchild
(b. 1937), cystic fibrosis specialist:
Cystic Fibrosis.

Professor Peter Goodfellow
(b. 1951), geneticist:
Gene Mapping.

Dr Len Goodwin
(1915–2008), researcher in the
chemotherapy of tropical diseases:
Africa.

Ms Shirley Goodwin
(b. 1947), public health specialist:
Public Health.

Professor Stewart Goodwin
(b. 1932), medical microbiologist:
Peptic Ulcer.

Professor David Gordon
(b. 1947), physician, Clinical Programme Director, Wellcome Trust:
ALSPAC, Clinical Pharmacology 1, Clinical Research, NATSAL.

Dr Ian Gould
(b. 1953), clinical microbiologist:
MRSA.

Dr Roy Goulding
(1916–2003), clinical toxicologist:
Safety of Drugs.

Professor John Govan
(b. 1942), microbiologist:
Cystic Fibrosis.

Sir James Gowans
(b. 1924), Secretary of the MRC:
Monoclonal Antibodies.

Professor David Grahame-Smith
(1933–2011), clinical pharmacologist:
Clinical Pharmacology 1, Clinical Pharmacology 2, Platinum Salts.

Professor Richard Gralla
(b. 1948), medical oncologist:
Platinum Salts.

Professor John Grange
(b. 1943), clinical microbiologist:
TB Chemotherapy.

Dr David Grant
(b. 1949), biochemist:
Leukaemia.

Professor Wyn Grant
(b. 1947), professor of politics:
Bovine TB.

Sir John Gray
(1918–2011), physiologist, Secretary of MRC:
Clinical Research, Monoclonal Antibodies.

Dr Winifred Gray
(b. 1937), cytopathologist:
Cervical Cancer.

Professor Jane Green
(b. 1943), medical geneticist:
Clinical Cancer Genetics.

Professor Irene Green
cellular biochemist:
Endogenous Opiates.

Professor Richard Green
(b. 1944), neuropharmacologist:
5-HT, Individual Interview.

Professor Trisha Greenhalgh
(b. 1959), primary care specialist:
Narrative Medicine.

Professor David Greenwood
(1935–2015), microbiologist:
MRSA, Post Penicillin.

Dr Roger Greenwood
(b. 1947), nephrologist:
Dialysis.

Dr Ian Gregg
(1925–2009), general practitioner:
Asthma.

Professor Richard Gregory
(1923–2010), experimental psychologist:
Applied Psychology, Individual Interview.

Professor John Griffin
(b. 1938), medical assessor to the Committee on Safety of Medicines:
Clinical Pharmacology 2.

Professor John Griffiths
(b. 1945), medical biochemist:
NMR and MRI.

Professor Rod Griffiths
(b. 1945), public health specialist:
Public Health.

Professor Jonathan Grigg
(b. 1957), respiratory paediatrician:
Air Pollution.

Professor John Groeger
(b. 1959), psychologist:
Applied Psychology.

Professor Jan Gronow
(b. 1945), waste management
academic:
Waste, Individual Interview.

Dr Geoffrey Guy
(b. 1954), industrial pharmacologist:
Cannabis.

Dr Jean Guy
(1941–2012), radiologist:
Medical Physics, Peptic Ulcer.

Professor Abe Guz
(1929–2014), physician:
Clinical Research.

Dr Djordje Gveric
(b. 1965), Director of the MS and
Parkinson's Tissue Bank:
Brain Banks.

Mrs Gill Gyte
(b. 1948), antenatal teacher:
Corticosteroids.

Mr John Haggith
(b. 1930), medical physicist:
Medical Physics.

Dr Angus Hall
(b. 1939), electronics engineer:
Ultrasound.

Mr Sherwin Hall
(1928–2014), veterinary surgeon:
Foot and Mouth.

Mr Stephen Hall
pharmacist, Ministry of Health:
Safety of Drugs.

Dr Nina Hallowell
(b. 1957), medical sociologist and
ethicist:
Ethics of Genetics.

Dr David Hamilton
(b. 1939), transplant surgeon and
medical historian:
Dialysis.

Professor John Hamilton
(b. 1937), gastroenterologist and
medical educator:
Rural Medicine.

Dr Patricia Hamilton
(b. 1951), neonatologist:
Neonatal Intensive Care.

Professor Jeremy Hamilton-Miller
(b. 1938), microbiologist:
MRSA.

Mrs Phyllis Hampson
(b. 1927), orthopaedic equipment
sales manager:
Hip Replacement.

Professor John Hampton
(b. 1937), cardiovascular physician:
Platelets.

Professor Alan Handyside
(b. 1951), developmental biologist,
reproductive specialist:
Genetic Testing.

Professor Geoffrey Hanks
(1946–2013), palliative care specialist:
Palliative Medicine.

Professor David Hannay
(b. 1939), GP:
General Practice.

Dr Stephen Hanney
(b. 1951), political scientist:
Corticosteroids.

Ms Helen Hanson
(b. 1950), Chair of SADA:
SAD.

Professor Lars Hanson
(b. 1934), paediatrician:
Breastfeeding.

Dr Peter Hanson
(b. 1949), biochemist:
Intestinal Absorption.

Professor Jane Harding
(b. 1955), neonatologist:
Corticosteroids.

Dr Kevin Hardinge
(b. 1939), orthopaedic surgeon:
Hip Replacement.

Dr Robin Harland
(1926–2012), former GP, lecturer in
sports medicine and medical historian:
Sports Medicine.

Professor David Harnden
(b. 1932), cancer geneticist:
Clinical Cancer Genetics.

Ms Christina Harocopos
(b. 1939), clinical nurse:
Clinical Cancer Genetics.

Professor (Sir) Peter Harper
(b. 1939), medical geneticist, policy
adviser, and historian of genetics:
*Clinical Cancer Genetics, Clinical
Genetics, Clinical Molecular Genetics,
Ethics of Genetics, Gene Mapping,
Genetic Testing, Rhesus Factor, Individual
Interview.*

Professor Kenneth Harrap
(b. 1931), oncological biochemist:
Platinum Salts.

Dr Hilary Harris
(b. 1943), GP:
Clinical Genetics.

Professor Rodney Harris
(b. 1932), medical geneticist:
Clinical Genetics, Genetic Testing.

Professor Michael Harrison
(b. 1936), neurologist:
Platelets.

Professor Roy Harrison
(b. 1948), environmental chemist:
Air Pollution.

Dr Philip Harrison-Read
(b. 1947), consultant psychiatrist:
Psychiatric Drugs.

Dr Julian Tudor Hart
(b. 1927), epidemiologist, GP:
*General Practice, Population-based
Research, Individual Interview.*

Dr Philip D'Arcy Hart
(1900–2006), physician, Director of
the MRC Tuberculosis Research Unit:
Population-based Research.

Sir Graham Hart
(b. 1940), civil servant at the
Department of Health:
NATSAL.

Professor David Harvey
(1936–2010), professor of paediatrics:
Neonatal Intensive Care.

Dr John Haybittle
(b. 1922), physicist:
Medical Physics.

Professor Frank Hayhoe
(1920–2009), haematologist:
Leukaemia.

Mr Graham Haynes
(b. 1950), intensive care nurse and
lecturer:
Intensive Care.

Professor Richard Hays
(b. 1953), rural GP and medical
educator:
Rural Medicine.

Dr John Hayward
(b. 1946), public health specialist:
Corticosteroids.

Professor David Healy
(b. 1954), psychiatrist:
Psychiatric Drugs.

Dr Vanessa Heggie
(b. 1978), medical/science historian:
Sports Medicine.

Dr Michael Hellier
(b. 1941), gastroenterologist:
Intestinal Absorption.

Dr Elisabet Helsing
(b. 1940), nutritional physiologist:
Breastfeeding.

Mr Nick Henderson
(b. 1926), veterinary surgeon:
Population-based Research.

Professor Ralph Hendrickse
(1926–2010), tropical paediatrician:
Africa.

Dr Leo Hepner
(1930–2015), management consultant
in biotechnology:
Post Penicillin.

Professor Stan Heptinstall
(b. 1946), biochemist:
Platelets.

Dr Amanda Herbert
(b. 1943), cytopathologist:
Cervical Cancer.

Councillor Lewis Herbert
(b. 1955), waste management historian
and local councillor:
Waste.

Dr Andrew Herxheimer
(1925–2016), pharmacologist, first
Chairman of the International Society
of Drug Bulletins:
*Clinical Pharmacology 1, Clinical
Pharmacology 2.*

Dr Edmund Hey
(1934–2009), paediatrician:
*Breastfeeding, Corticosteroids, Maternal
Care.*

Mr Mike Heywood-Waddington
(b. 1929), orthopaedic surgeon:
Hip Replacement.

Mrs Eleanor Hickie
(b. 1939), nurse and Asthmatic:
Asthma.

Dr Peter Higgins
(b. 1926), virologist:
Common Cold Unit.

Mr Russell Higgins
(b. 1954), electronic engineer:
NIMR.

Professor Roger Higgs
(b. 1943), former President of the
London Medical Group:
Medical Ethics.

Mr Gordon Higson
(1932–2001), former Director of the
Scientific and Technical Branch of the
Department of Health and Social
Security:
NMR and MRI.

Mr Barry Hill
(b. 1948), educationist:
Sports Medicine.

Professor Ray Hill
(b. 1945), pharmacologist:
Clinical Pharmacology 2.

Dr Richard Hillier
(b. 1940), palliative care specialist:
Palliative Medicine.

Dr Elizabeth Hills
(b. 1935), consultant physician:
TB Chemotherapy.

Professor Richard Himsworth
(b. 1937), physician:
Clinical Research.

Professor Graham Hitch
(b. 1946), psychologist:
Applied Psychology.

Professor Michael Hobsley
(b. 1929), surgeon:
Peptic Ulcer, Sports Medicine.

Dr Kay Hocking
(b. 1913), entomologist:
Africa.

Dr Clare Hodges
(1957–2011), pseudonym of Mrs
Elizabeth (Liz) Brice, founding
member of the Alliance for Cannabis
Therapeutics:
Cannabis.

Dr Keith Hodgkin
(1918–1999), GP:
General Practice.

Professor Shirley Hodgson
(b. 1945), consultant geneticist:
*Clinical Cancer Genetics, Clinical
Genetics, Ethics of Genetics, Muscular
Dystrophy, Individual Interview.*

Dr Nicholas Hoenich
(b. 1946), medical technologist:
Dialysis.

Dr James Hoeschele
(b. 1937), pharmaceutical chemist:
Platinum Salts.

Professor Victor Hoffbrand
(b. 1935), haematologist:
Leukaemia.

Sir Raymond Hoffenberg
(1923–2007), physician:
Clinical Research.

Dr Eric Hoffman
(b. 1958), geneticist:
Muscular Dystrophy.

Dr David Hogg
(b. 1981), rural GP:
Rural Medicine.

Dr Anita Holdcroft
(b. 1947), anaesthetist, pain researcher:
Cannabis.

Mrs Cathy Holding
(b. 1957), laboratory research assistant:
Genetic Testing.

Dr Derek Holdsworth
(b. 1933), physiologist:
Intestinal Absorption.

Professor Stephen Holgate
(b. 1947), immunopharmacologist:
Asthma.

Professor Walter Holland
(b. 1929), epidemiologist:
Public Health.

Dr Arthur Hollman
(1923–2014), cardiologist, historian of
medicine:
Cholesterol, Heart Transplant, Platelets.

Mr Roger Hooper
(b. 1944), lab technician:
NIMR.

Professor John Hopewell
(1920–2015), urological surgeon:
Dialysis.

Dr Tom Hopwood
(b. 1919), tropical medicine expert:
Africa.

Dr John Horder
(1919–2012), GP, President of the
RCGP:
General Practice.

Sir Godfrey Hounsfield
(1919–2004), engineer, Nobel
Laureate:
NMR and MRI.

Dr Sheila Howarth (Lady McMichael)
(1920–2000), Principal Medical Officer
– Medical Research Council:
*Africa, Clinical Research, Common Cold
Unit, Haemophilia, Population-based
Research.*

Professor Jack Howell
(1926–2015), consultant physician:
Asthma.

Professor Peter Howie
(b. 1939), obstetrician and
gynaecologist:
Breastfeeding.

Ross Howie
(b. 1933), neonatal paediatrician:
Corticosteroids.

Dr Andrew Hoy
(b. 1949), clinical oncologist, consultant
in palliative medicine:
Palliative Medicine.

Professor Daniel Hoyer
(b. 1954), pharmacologist:
5-HT.

Professor Geoffrey Hudson
(b. 1962) medical historian:
Rural Medicine.

Professor Anne Hudson Jones
(b. 1944), medical humanities scholar:
Narrative Medicine.

Dr Philip Hugh-Jones
(1917–2010), respiratory physician:
*Population-based Research, Individual
Interview.*

Mrs Janie Hughes
(b. 1944), interviewer and fieldworker:
Population-based Research, Individual Interview.

Dr Jeff Hughes
historian of science:
Medical Physics.

Professor John Hughes,
pharmacologist:
Endogenous Opiates.

Dr Nevin Hughes-Jones
(b. 1923), haematologist:
Rhesus Factor.

Professor Sir David Hull
(b. 1932), consultant paediatrician:
Neonatal Intensive Care.

Professor Maj Hultén, molecular geneticist:
Gene Mapping.

Miss Tracy Humberstone
(b. 1964), cystic fibrosis patient and healthcare consultant:
Cystic Fibrosis.

Professor Patrick Humphrey
(b. 1946), industrial pharmacologist:
5-HT, Migraine, Individual Interview.

Professor Steve Humphries
(b. 1950), cardiovascular geneticist:
Cholesterol.

Dr Jackie Hunter
pharmacologist:
5-HT.

Dr Kenneth Hunter
(1939–2013), consultant physician:
Clinical Pharmacology 1.

Dr Peter Hunter
(b. 1938), consultant physician, endocrinologist:
Applied Psychology, Cystic Fibrosis, Environmental Toxicology, Leukaemia, Maternal Care, Pain, Peptic Ulcer, Platelets, Rhesus Factor.

Professor Brian Hurwitz
(b. 1951), medical humanities scholar:
Migraine, Narrative Medicine.

Dr O A N (Nasseem) Husain
(1924–2014), cytopathologist:
Cervical Cancer.

Ms Victoria Hutchins
(b. 1977), multiple sclerosis patient:
Cannabis.

Dr Michael Hutson
(b. 1942), sports medicine specialist:
Sports Medicine.

Professor Michael Hutt
(1922–2000), tropical pathologist:
Africa.

Professor Peter Hutton
(b. 1947), consultant anaesthetist:
Intensive Care.

Mrs Yasmin Iles-Caven
(b. 1962), Departmental manager for ALSPAC:
ALSPAC.

Professor Victor Inem
(b. 1955), professor of family medicine:
Rural Medicine.

Professor Ilsley Ingram
(1919–2004), haematologist:
Haemophilia.

Professor Bill Inman
(1929–2005), medical civil servant:
Safety of Drugs, Individual Interview.

Professor James Ironside
(b. 1954), neuropathologist:
Brain Banks.

Dr Craig Irvine
(b. 1958), narrative medicine and
medical humanities scholar:
Narrative Medicine.

Professor Ian Isherwood
(b. 1931), neuroradiologist:
NMR and MRI.

Professor Leslie Iversen
(b. 1937), pharmacologist:
Cannabis, Endogenous Opiates.

Sir David Jack
(1924–2011), industrial
pharmacologist:
Asthma.

Dr Anthony Jackson
(1918–2005), consultant paediatrician:
Cystic Fibrosis.

Professor Mark Jackson
medical historian:
Asthma.

Professor Pat Jacobs
(b. 1934), cytogeneticist:
Clinical Molecular Genetics.

Dr Bobbie Jacobson
(b. 1950), public health physician:
NATSAL.

Professor Margot Jefferys
(1916–1999), medical sociologist:
General Practice.

Mrs Rosemary Jenkins
(b. 1942), administrator for Royal
College of Midwives:
Maternal Care.

Professor David Jenkins
(b. 1946), pathologist:
Cervical Cancer.

Dr Tony Jenkins
(b. 1936), clinical immunologist:
TB Chemotherapy.

Dr Joanna Jenkinson
(b. 1977), MRC Programme Manger:
Brain Banks.

Professor Alec Jenner
(1927–2014), psychiatrist:
Psychiatric Drugs.

Professor Bryan Jennett
(1926–2008), neurosurgeon:
Medical Ethics.

Dr (William) Alan Jennings
(1923–2016), medical physicist:
Medical Physics.

Dr David Jewell
(b. 1950), GP obstetrician:
Maternal Care.

Dr Amina Jindani
(b. 1936), coordinator of clinical trials
in TB therapeutics:
TB Chemotherapy.

Professor Dame Anne Johnson
(b. 1954), Principal Investigator on
the 1990, 2000 and 2010 National
Surveys of Sexual Attitudes and
Lifestyles:
Cervical Cancer, NATSAL.

Dr Jeremy Johnson
(b. 1950), hospice medical director:
Pain.

Mr Stanley Johnson
(b. 1940), former MEP, Head of the
European Commission's Prevention of
Pollution and Nuisances division:
Environmental Toxicology.

Dr Alan Johnston
(1928–2012), clinical geneticist:
Clinical Genetics.

Dr Belinda Johnston
(b. 1957), gastrointestinal researcher:
Peptic Ulcer.

Ms Emma Jones
(b. 1974), medical historian:
Bovine TB.

Mr Ian Jones
(b. 1965), publisher:
Corticosteroids.

Ms Marion Jones
epidemiological field worker:
*Population-based Research, Individual
Interview.*

Dr Peter Jones
(b. 1937), consultant paediatrician,
director of haemophilia centre:
Haemophilia.

Dr Richard Jones
(b. 1943), chemical pathologist:
ALSPAC.

Professor Roger Jones
(b. 1948), GP, professor of general
practice:
Peptic Ulcer.

Professor Terry Jones, physicist:
Individual Interview.

Professor Trevor Jones
(b. 1942), pharmacology research
director:
Clinical Pharmacology 1, Migraine.

Mr David Joranson
(b. 1941), physician:
Pain.

Dr Tony Jordan
(b. 1931), entomologist:
Africa.

Dr Simon Joseph
(b. 1940), cardiologist:
Heart Transplant.

Professor Ian Judson
(b. 1951), medical oncologist:
Platinum Salts.

Professor Desmond Julian
(b. 1926), cardiologist and
pharmacologist:
Platelets.

Professor Joachim Kalden
(b. 1937), clinical immunologist:
TNF.

Dr Leon Kaufman
(b. 1927), anaesthetist:
Pain.

Professor Alberto Kaumann
(b. 1936), pharmacologist:
5-HT.

Dr Clifford Kay
(b. 1927), GP:
General Practice.

Dr Humphrey Kay
(1923–2009), haematologist:
Leukaemia.

Dr Angela Kearns
(b. 1959), microbiologist:
MRSA.

Dr Lloyd Kemp
(b. 1914), physicist:
Medical Physics.

Professor Sir Ian Kennedy
(b. 1941), lawyer and ethicist:
Medical Ethics.

Professor David Kerr
(1927–2014), professor of renal
medicine:
Dialysis.

Mrs Ann Kershaw
(b. 1949), genetic nurse counsellor:
Clinical Genetics.

Mrs Lauren Kerzin–Storrar
(b. 1955), genetic counsellor:
Clinical Genetics.

Professor Stewart Kilpatrick
(1925–2013), epidemiologist:
*Population-based Research, Individual
Interview.*

Mr Geoff King
(b. 1947), orthopaedic technician:
Hip Replacement.

Mr Raymond Kirk
(b. 1923), consultant surgeon:
Peptic Ulcer.

Mr John Kirkup
(b. 1928), orthopaedic surgeon and
surgical historian:
Hip Replacement.

Dr Georges Köhler
(1946–1995), immunologist, Nobel
Laureate:
Monoclonal Antibodies.

Dr Felix Konotey-Ahulu
(b. 1930), consultant physician and
geneticist:
Dialysis.

Professor Leopold Koss
(1920–2012), cytopathologist:
Cervical Cancer.

Dr Oleg Kravtchenko
(b. 1963), rural GP:
Rural Medicine.

Dr Ekke Kuenssberg
(1913–2000), GP, President of the
RCGP:
Safety of Drugs.

Professor Parveen Kumar
(b. 1942), gastroenterologist:
Clinical Pharmacology 2.

Dr Suresh Kumar
(b. 1961), consultant in palliative
medicine:
Pain.

Dr Belinda Kumpel
(b. 1948), haematology research
scientist:
Rhesus Factor.

Mr Krishna (Ravi) Kunzru
(b. 1937), orthopaedic surgeon:
Hip Replacement.

Professor Sir Peter Lachmann
(b. 1931), immunologist:
Autoimmunity, Clinical Research.

Professor Harold Lambert
(1926–2017), infectious diseases
professor:
Post Penicillin.

Dr Donald Lane
(b. 1935), consultant chest physician:
Asthma.

Professor Michael Langman
(1935–2014), gastroenterologist:
Peptic Ulcer.

Professor Peter Lantos
(b. 1939), neuropathologist:
Brain Banks.

Dr John Launer
(b. 1949), GP and family therapist:
Narrative Medicine.

Professor Desmond Laurence
(b. 1922), pharmacologist:
Clinical Pharmacology 1.

Professor Michael Laurence
(b. 1924), clinical geneticist:
Clinical Genetics.

Dr John Law
(b. 1935), medical physicist:
Medical Physics.

Mr Laz Lazarou
(b. 1962), medical geneticist:
Clinical Molecular Genetics.

Dr James Le Fanu
(b. 1950), GP, medical journalist:
Psychiatric Drugs.

Professor Iain Ledingham
(b. 1935), surgeon, intensive care
consultant:
Intensive Care.

Miss Betty Lee
(b. 1925), orthopaedic nurse:
Hip Replacement.

Professor Christine Lee
(b. 1943), consultant haematologist:
Haemophilia.

Professor Alan Lehmann
(b. 1946), molecular geneticist:
Clinical Cancer Genetics.

Professor John Lennard-Jones
(b. 1927), consultant
gastroenterologist:
Peptic Ulcer.

Professor Maurice Lessof
(b. 1924), physician and clinical
immunologist:
Autoimmunity, Heart Transplant.

Mr Alan Lettin
(b. 1931), orthopaedic surgeon:
Hip Replacement.

Professor Roy Levin
(b. 1935), physiologist:
Intestinal Absorption.

Dr Mark Levy
(b. 1948), general practioner:
Asthma.

Dr Peter Lewis
(b. 1944), industrial pharmacologist:
Clinical Pharmacology 2.

Professor Alfred Lewy
(b. 1945), psychiatrist:
SAD.

Dr Owen Lidwell
(1914–2010), external scientific staff
member for Medical Research Council
at Common Cold Unit:
Common Cold Unit.

Professor Sidney Liebowitz,
immunologist:
Autoimmunity.

Professor Sir Graham (Mont) Liggins
(1926–2010), obstetrician and gynaecologist:
Corticosteroids

Professor Richard Lilford
(b. 1950), consultant obstetrician and gynaecologist/epidemiologist:
Corticosteroids.

Professor Sir John Lilleyman
(b. 1945), consultant haematologist:
Leukaemia.

Professor Gerald Lincoln
(b. 1945), chronobiologist:
SAD.

Dr James Littlewood
(b. 1932), consultant paediatrician, former Chairman of the UK Cystic Fibrosis Trust:
Cystic Fibrosis.

Dr Stephen Lock
(b. 1929), editor of the British Medical Journal (1975–1991):
Endogenous Opiates, General Practice, Medical Ethics, Safety of Drugs.

Dr Eunice Lockey
(b. 1925), clinical pathologist:
Heart Transplant.

Dr Robert Logan
(b. 1959), gastroenterologist:
Peptic Ulcer.

Professor Robert Logie
(b. 1954), psychologist:
Applied Psychology.

Professor Donald Longmore
(b. 1928), consultant surgeon and clinical physiologist:
Heart Transplant, NMR and MRI.

Mr Philip Lord
(b. 1945), bioinformatician:
Air Pollution, Individual Interview.

Professor Monty Losowsky
(b. 1931), emeritus professor of medicine:
Dialysis, Sports Medicine.

Dr Irvine Loudon
(1924–2015), GP, medical historian:
General Practice, Maternal Care.

Professor Seth Love
(b. 1955), neuropathologist:
Brain Banks.

Professor James Lovelock
(b. 1919), member of scientific staff at the National Institute for Medical Research:
Common Cold Unit, Environmental Toxicology.

Professor Gordon Lowe
(b. 1949), consultant physician:
Cholesterol.

Professor Rob Lucas
(b. 1968), neurobiologist:
SAD.

Professor Anneke Lucassen
(b. 1962), clinical geneticist:
Ethics of Genetics.

Dr Brandon Lush
(b. 1920), Principal Medical Officer – Medical Research Council:
Applied Psychology, Clinical Research.

Professor Domhnall MacAuley
(b. 1957), professor of primary health care:
Sports Medicine.

Dr Peter MacCallum
(b. 1958), haematologist:
Platelets.

Dr Anita MacDonald
(b. 1956), paediatric dietician:
Cystic Fibrosis.

Professor David Macdonald
(b. 1951), ecologist:
Bovine TB.

Dr Fiona Macdonald
(b. 1954), molecular geneticist:
Clinical Molecular Genetics.

Mrs Rose Macdonald
(b. 1930), physiotherapist and director of physiotherapy for the London Marathon (1981–2005):
Sports Medicine.

Professor Alison Macfarlane
(b. 1942), medical statistician:
Air Pollution, Maternal Care, Individual Interview.

Professor Anne MacGregor
(b. 1960), specialist in headache and women's health:
Migraine.

Dr Judith Mackay
(b. 1943), physician, senior policy adviser to the WHO:
Tobacco Control.

Dr Elizabeth Mackenzie
(b. 1934), cytopathologist:
Cervical Cancer.

Mr Ian MacKenzie
(b. 1942), obstetrician and gynaecologist:
Rhesus Factor.

Professor Allan Maclean
(b. 1947), obstetrician and gynaecologist:
Maternal Care.

Professor Ian MacLennan
(b. 1939), immunologist:
Leukaemia.

Professor Donald Macleod
(b. 1941), former President of the British Association of Sports and Exercise Medicine:
Sports Medicine.

Professor Patrick MacLeod
(b. 1940), medical geneticist:
Individual Interview.

Dr Joan Macnab, geneticist:
Cervical Cancer.

Professor Jane Macnaughton
(b. 1960), medical historian:
Narrative Medicine.

Sir Malcolm Macnaughton
(1925–2016), obstetrician and gynaecologist:
Medical Ethics.

Professor John MacVicar
(1927–2011), obstetrician and gynaecologist:
Ultrasound.

Ms Susan Madge
nurse consultant:
Cystic Fibrosis.

Dr Martyn Mahaut-Smith
(b. 1962), physiologist:
Platelets.

Professor Eamonn Maher
(b. 1956), consultant geneticist:
Clinical Cancer Genetics.

Professor Jane Maher
(b. 1953), clinical oncologist:
Palliative Medicine.

Professor Chris Main
(b. 1947), clinical psychologist:
Pain.

Professor Sir Ravinder Nath (Tiny) Maini
(b. 1937), rheumatologist:
TNF.

Professor Sue Malcolm
(d. 2015), molecular geneticist:
Gene Mapping, Genetic Testing.

Professor John Mallard
(b. 1927), medical physicist:
Medical Physics, NMR and MRI.

Professor Sir Netar Mallick
(b. 1935), renal physician:
Dialysis.

Dr Maureen Malowany
(b. 1949), medical historian:
Africa.

Professor David Mann
(b. 1948), neuropathologist:
Brain Banks.

Professor Sir Peter Mansfield
(1933–2017), physicist, Nobel Laureate:
NMR and MRI, Individual Interview.

Professor Tim Mant
(b. 1954), pharmacologist:
Clinical Pharmacology 2.

Dr Diana Manuel
medical historian:
Medical Ethics.

Dr Marshall Marinker
(b. 1930), GP, medical educator:
General Practice.

Professor Isaac Marks
(b. 1935), psychiatrist:
Psychiatric Drugs.

Professor Vincent Marks
(b. 1930), biochemist:
Cholesterol.

Professor Hilary Marland
medical historian:
Maternal Care.

Professor Charles Marsden
(b. 1943), pharmacologist:
5-HT, Individual Interview.

Dr Frank Marsh
(1936–2011), nephrologist:
Dialysis.

Mr Jonathan Marsh
(b. 1942), head of department of engineering at NIMR:
NIMR, Individual Interview.

Professor William Marslen-Wilson
(b. 1945), psychologist:
Applied Psychology.

Professor Adrian Martineau
(b. 1971), TB researcher:
TB Chemotherapy.

Dr Edwin Massey
(b. 1966), haematologist:
Rhesus Factor.

Mr Ian Mathison
(b. 1932), lab technician:
NIMR.

Dr James Matthews
(b. 1930), research scientist in blood
coagulation:
Haemophilia.

Professor Robert Maynard
(b. 1951), physiologist, medical civil
servant:
Air Pollution, Environmental Toxicology.

Dr Paul McCarthy
(b. 1942), physician:
Asthma.

Professor Glenn McCluggage
(b. 1963), histopathologist:
Cervical Cancer.

Professor Kenneth McColl
(b. 1950), consultant
gastroenterologist:
Peptic Ulcer.

Dr James McCracken
(b. 1930), GP:
Asthma.

Professor Denis McDevitt
(b. 1937), clinical pharmacologist:
*Clinical Pharmacology 1, Clinical
Pharmacology 2.*

Professor Norman McDicken
(b. 1940), medical physicist:
Ultrasound.

Professor W Ian McDonald
(1933–2006), consultant neurologist,
medical historian:
Autoimmunity, Clinical Research.

Dr Gordon McGlone
(b. 1951), CEO of Gloucestershire
Wildlife Trust:
Bovine TB.

Professor Sir Ian McGregor
(1922–2007), malariologist:
Africa.

Professor Neil McIntosh
(b. 1942), neonatologist:
Neonatal Intensive Care.

Professor Joe McKie
(b. 1925), clinical physicist:
Medical Physics.

Dr Faith McLellan
(b. 1960), medical journalist:
Tobacco Control.

Professor Peter McLeod
(b. 1946), psychologist:
Applied Psychology.

Dr Margaret McNay
(b. 1945), obstetrician and
gynaecologist:
Ultrasound.

Professor Alan McNeilly
(b. 1947), endocrinologist:
Breastfeeding.

Dr Iain McNicol
(b. 1949), rural GP:
Rural Medicine.

Professor Klim McPherson
(b. 1941), public heath epidemiologist:
Public Health.

Professor Thomas Meade
(b. 1936), Director of the MRC Epidemiology and Medical Care Unit:
General Practice, Platelets.

Dr Jeanette Meadway
(b. 1947), consultant physician:
TB Chemotherapy.

Dr Margaret Mearns
(1924–2010), paediatrician:
Cystic Fibrosis.

Professor Raphael Mechoulam
(b. 1930), pharmacologist:
Cannabis.

Mr Keith Meldrum
(b. 1937), Chief Veterinary Officer:
Bovine TB, Foot and Mouth.

Dr Catherine Mercer
(b. 1974), statistician:
NATSAL.

Dr Linda Meredith
(b. 1955), medical geneticist:
Clinical Molecular Genetics.

Professor David Metcalfe
(b. 1930), GP:
General Practice.

Dr Richard Meyer
(b. 1946), ecologist:
Bovine TB.

Dr William (Bill) Miall
(1917–2004), scientific staff member of MRC Pneumoconiosis Research Unit:
General Practice, Population-based Research, Individual Interview.

Professor Kim Michaelsen
(b. 1948), paediatric nutritionist:
Breastfeeding.

Dr Helen Middleton–Price
(b. 1955), molecular geneticist:
Clinical Molecular Genetics.

Professor Anthony Miller
(b. 1931), clinical epidemiologist:
Cervical Cancer.

Dr Paul Miller
(b. 1940), gastroenterologist:
Cholesterol.

Mrs Riva Miller
(b. 1935), social worker:
Haemophilia.

Professor Tony Milner
(b. 1938), neonatologist:
Asthma.

Professor César Milstein
(1927–2002), molecular biologist, immunologist, Nobel Laureate:
Monoclonal Antibodies.

Mr Wesley Miner
(b. 1948), industrial pharmacologist:
5-HT, Platinum Salts, Individual Interview.

Dr George Misiewicz
(b. 1930), gastroenterologist:
Peptic Ulcer.

Dr David Misselbrook
(b. 1956), GP:
Medical Ethics.

Professor Ross Mitchell
(1920–2006), paediatrician:
Asthma, Neonatal Intensive Care.

Professor Denis (Denny) Mitchison
(b. 1919), bacteriologist:
Post Penicillin, TB Chemotherapy.

Professor Ursula Mittwoch
(b. 1924), geneticist:
Clinical Genetics, Genetic Testing.

Professor Bernadette Modell
(b. 1935), geneticist, thalassaemia
specialist:
*Clinical Molecular Genetics, Ethics of
Genetics, Genetic Testing.*

Professor Michael Modell
(b. 1937) GP:
Clinical Genetics.

Professor Anthony Moffat
(b. 1942), pharmaceutical analyst:
Cannabis.

Dr Pål Møller
(b. 1946), cancer geneticist:
Clinical Cancer Genetics.

Professor Patrick Mollison
(b. 1914), haematologist:
Rhesus Factor.

Professor Sir Salvador Moncada
(b. 1944), research pharmacologist:
Platelets, Individual Interview.

Professor Dame Barbara Monroe
(b. 1951), social worker and hospital
chief executive:
Palliative Medicine.

Mr John Montague
(b. 1952), MAFF veterinary officer:
Bovine TB.

Professor Kathryn Montgomery
(b. 1939), medical humanities scholar:
Narrative Medicine.

The Duke of Montrose
(b. 1935), livestock farmer:
Foot and Mouth.

Dr Catherine Moody
(b. 1957), MRC programme manager:
Brain Banks.

Dr John Moore-Gillon
(b. 1953), consultant chest physician:
TB Chemotherapy.

Mrs Hilary Morgan
(b. 1935), lab technician:
NIMR.

Professor Jennifer Morgan
cell biologist:
Muscular Dystrophy.

Professor Michael Morgan
(b. 1942), programme director,
Wellcome Trust:
Gene Mapping.

Professor David Morrell
(b. 1925), GP:
General Practice.

Professor Howard Morris
biochemist:
Endogenous Opiates.

Mr James Morris
(b. 1929), veterinary officer with
MAFF:
Foot and Mouth.

Professor Jerry Morris
(1910–2009), epidemiologist:
Cholesterol.

Dr Peter Morris
(b. 1956), historian of chemistry:
NIMR.

Dr Harry Morrow Brown
(1917–2013), consultant chest
physician:
Asthma.

Professor David Morton
(b. 1943), medical ethicist:
Medical Ethics.

Dr Ornella Moscucci
(b. 1954), medical historian:
Public Health.

Dr Noel Mowat
(1927–2010), veterinary vaccinologist:
Foot and Mouth.

Professor Miranda Mugford
(b. 1950), health economist:
Corticosteroids.

Dame Lorna Muirhead
(b. 1942), midwife:
Maternal Care.

Mrs Brenda Mullinger
(b. 1949), clinical trials coordinator:
Corticosteroids.

Ms Kathryn (Kathy) Mulvey
(b. 1966), public health advocate:
Tobacco Control.

Mrs Elizabeth Mumford
(b. 1958), lecturer in medical law:
ALSPAC, Ethics of Genetics.

Professor Donald Munro
(1925–2013), professor of medicine:
Clinical Research.

Professor Francesco Muntoni
(b. 1959), paediatric neurologist:
Muscular Dystrophy.

Mr David J Murnaghan
(b. 1938), physicist:
Medical Physics.

Baroness Elaine Murphy
(b. 1947), psychiatrist:
Psychiatric Drugs.

Dr Shaun Murphy
(b. 1951), medical administrator and
historian:
Population-based Research.

Dr Nicolas (Nick) Myant
(b. 1917), clinical biochemist:
Cholesterol.

Professor Richard Naftalin
(b. 1939), physiologist:
Intestinal Absorption.

Sir Patrick Nairne
(1921–2013), civil servant, Permanent
Secretary of the Department of
Health and Social Security:
Clinical Research.

Ms Brenda Nally
(b. 1941), outreach officer, UK Brain
Bank for Autism:
Brain Banks.

Professor Robert Naylor
(b. 1943), pharmacologist:
Platinum Salts.

Ms Kay Neale
(b. 1946), polyposis registry manager
and research coordinator:
*Clinical Cancer Genetics, Individual
Interview.*

Dr Francis Neary
(b. 1971), medical historian:
Hip Replacement.

Professor George Nelson
(1923–2009), parasitologist:
Africa.

Professor Andy Ness
(b. 1962), epidemiologist:
Population-based Research.

Mr John Newell
science journalist:
Monoclonal Antibodies.

Professor Angela Newing
(b. 1938), medical physicist:
Medical Physics.

Dr Bill Newsom
(b. 1932), microbiologist:
MRSA.

Dr Alice Nicholls
(b. 1975), medical historian:
Intensive Care.

Dr Alex Nicholson
(b. 1970), specialist in palliative
medicine:
Pain.

Dr Richard Nicholson
founder, Chairman of the Association
of Research Ethics Committees
(UK):
Medical Ethics.

Professor Malcolm Nicolson
(b. 1952), medical historian:
Ultrasound.

Dr Haik Nikogosian
(b. 1955), WHO secretariat:
Tobacco Control.

Professor Walter Nimmo
(b. 1947), clinical pharmacologist:
Clinical Pharmacology 1.

Dr Bill Noble
(b. 1956), palliative care specialist:
Palliative Medicine.

Dr Archie Norman
(1912–2016), paediatrician, Chairman
of the Medical Advisory Committee of
the Cystic Fibrosis Research Trust:
Asthma, Cystic Fibrosis, Rhesus Factor.

Professor Colin Normand
(1928–2011), paediatrician:
Neonatal Intensive Care.

Dr Keith Norris
(b. 1928), biophysicist:
Individual Interview

Dr Robin Norris
(1931–2015), cardiologist:
Platelets.

Professor Alan North
(b. 1944), neuropharmacologist:
Individual Interview.

Professor Timothy Northfield
(1935–2008), consultant
gastroenterologist:
Peptic Ulcer.

Dr Jean Northover
(b. 1928), scientist, parent of dialysis
patient:
Dialysis.

Dr William Notcutt
(b. 1946), neurologist:
Cannabis, Palliative Medicine.

Dr Andrew Nunn
(b. 1943), statistician:
TB Chemotherapy, Individual Interview.

Dr Michael O'Brien
(b. 1938), neurologist:
Migraine.

Professor Moira O'Brien
(b. 1933), consultant in osteoporosis
and sports medicine:
Sports Medicine.

Professor Chris O'Callaghan
(b. 1959), paediatrician:
Asthma.

Mrs Rachel O'Leary
(b. 1949), breastfeeding counsellor:
Breastfeeding.

Professor Colm Ó'Moráin
(b. 1946), gastroenterologist:
Peptic Ulcer.

Professor Ann Oakley
(b. 1944), sociologist:
Corticosteroids.

Dr Chisholm Ogg
(b. 1938), nephrologist:
Dialysis.

Dr Ahmed Ezra Ogwell
(b. 1969), Kenyan civil servant:
Tobacco Control.

Dr John Old
(b. 1949), haematologist:
Clinical Molecular Genetics.

Mr John Older
(b. 1935), orthopaedic surgeon:
Hip Replacement.

Professor Jes Olesen
(b. 1941), neurologist:
Migraine.

Professor Michael Oliver
(1925–2015), cardiologist:
Cholesterol, Platelets.

Professor Tom Oppé
(1925–2007), paediatrician:
Neonatal Intensive Care.

Professor Roger Ordidge
(b. 1956), physicist:
Individual Interview

Professor Michael Orme
(b. 1940), clinical pharmacologist:
*Clinical Pharmacology 1, Clinical
Pharmacology 2.*

**Professor Lawrence (Peter)
Ormerod**
(b. 1950), chest physician:
TB Chemotherapy.

Dr Sidney Osborn
(b. 1918), medical physicist:
Medical Physics.

Dr Knut Øvreberg
(1928–2012), chest physician:
TB Chemotherapy.

Dr David Owen
journalist:
Monoclonal Antibodies.

Dr Alec Oxford
(b. 1940), chemist:
Migraine.

Professor Chris Packard
(b. 1953), physician:
Cholesterol.

Professor Clive Page
(b. 1958), pharmacologist:
Platelets.

Professor Lesley Page
(b. 1944), midwife:
Maternal Care.

Ms Gabrielle Palmer
(b. 1947), public health nutritionist:
Breastfeeding.

Dr Ingar Palmlund
(b. 1938), medical sociologist:
Environmental Toxicology.

Professor Michael Parker
(b. 1958), medical ethicist:
Ethics of Genetics.

Dr Colin Murray Parkes
(b. 1928), psychiatrist:
Pain, Palliative Medicine.

Professor Sir Eldryd Parry
(b. 1930), physician and medical
educator:
*Africa, Rural Medicine, Individual
Interview.*

Dr John Lloyd Parry
(b. 1936), GP:
Sports Medicine.

Professor Terence A Partridge
(b. 1940), cell biologist:
Muscular Dystrophy.

Mr Nick Patterson
(b. 1946), contract manager of refuse
collection:
Waste.

Dr John Paulley
(1918–2007), gastroenterologist:
Peptic Ulcer.

Miss Lesley Pavitt
(b. 1944), dialysis nurse:
Dialysis.

Dr Brian Payne
(b. 1945), consultant physician:
Medical Ethics.

Professor Malcolm Peaker
(b. 1943), physiologist:
Breastfeeding.

Sir Stanley Peart
(b. 1922), physician, Trustee of the
Wellcome Trust:
*Clinical Research, General Practice,
NATSAL, Platelets.*

Dr Richard Peatfield
(b. 1949), consultant neurologist:
Migraine.

Dr Anthony Peck
(b. 1933), industrial clinical
pharmacologist:
*Clinical Pharmacology 1, Clinical
Pharmacology 2.*

Professor Catherine Peckham
(b. 1937), paediatric epidemiologist:
ALSPAC.

Mr Roger Peel
(b. 1935), obstetrician and
gynaecologist:
Maternal Care.

Dr Tanja Pekez-Pavlisko
(b. 1961), emergency medicine
physician:
Rural Medicine.

Professor John Pemberton
(1912–2010), professor of social and
preventative medicine:
Population-based Research.

Professor Marcus Pembrey
(b. 1943), paediatrician and clinical
geneticist:
*ALSPAC, Clinical Genetics, Ethics of
Genetics, Genetic Testing, Individual
Interview.*

Professor Brian Pentecost
(1934–2015), cardiologist:
Platelets.

Professor Sir Denis Pereira Gray
(b. 1935), GP:
Rural Medicine.

Professor Hugh Perry
(b. 1952), neuropathologist:
Brain Banks.

Dr Mark Perry
GP:
General Practice.

Professor Roger Pertwee
(b. 1942), pharmacologist:
Cannabis.

Professor Timothy Peters
(b. 1939), clinical biochemist:
Intestinal Absorption.

Professor Wallace Peters
(b. 1924), protozoologist:
Africa.

Professor Julian Peto
(b. 1945), oncological epidemiologist:
Cervical Cancer.

Professor Judith Petts
(b. 1954), waste management and
environmental scientist:
Waste, Individual Interview.

Professor Naomi Pfeffer
(b. 1946), medical historian:
Genetic Testing.

Mr Elliot Philipp
(1915–2010), obstetrician and
gynaecologist:
Maternal Care, Rhesus Factor.

Professor Ian Phillips
(b. 1936), medical microbiologist:
MRSA.

Professor Robin Phillips
(b. 1952), surgeon:
Clinical Cancer Genetics.

Professor Brian Pickering
(b. 1936), neuroendocrinologist,
deputy Vice–Chancellor, University of
Bristol:
ALSPAC.

Professor John Pickstone
(1944–2014), medical historian:
Dialysis, Hip Replacement.

Dr Catherine Pike
(1920–2016), cytopathologist:
Cervical Cancer.

Dr Gordon Piller
(1925–2005), former Director of the
Leukaemia Research Fund:
Leukaemia.

Dr Andrew Pinder
(b. 1953), medical physicist and
engineer:
NIMR, Individual Interview.

Dr Malcolm Pines
(b. 1925), psychiatrist:
Psychiatric Drugs.

Dr Tyrone Pitt
(b. 1948), microbiologist:
MRSA.

Dr Hugh Platt
(b. 1921), veterinary pathologist:
Foot and Mouth.

Dr Margaret Platts
(b. 1924), consultant nephrologist:
Dialysis.

Professor John Playfair
immunologist:
Autoimmunity.

Dr Walter Plowright
(1923–2010), veterinary microbiologist:
Foot and Mouth.

Lord Plumb
(b. 1927), farmer and politician:
Foot and Mouth.

Professor Stuart Pocock
medical statistician:
Cholesterol.

Professor Paul Polani
(1914–2006), geneticist and
paediatrician:
Genetic Testing.

Dr Jon Pollock
(b. 1948), epidemiologist:
ALSPAC.

Mr Richard Porter
(b. 1951), obstetrician and
gynaecologist:
Maternal Care.

Mrs Betty Porterfield
scientific staff at Common Cold Unit:
Common Cold Unit.

Dr James Porterfield
(1924–2010), member of the scientific
staff at the MRC Common Cold Unit:
Common Cold Unit.

Dr Martina Pötschke-Langer
(b. 1951), public health activist and
WHO adviser:
Tobacco Control.

Professor Roy Pounder
(b. 1944), gastroenterologist:
Intestinal Absorption, Peptic Ulcer.

Professor Sue Povey
(b. 1942), human geneticist:
*Clinical Genetics, Gene Mapping, Genetic
Testing.*

Professor Ray Powles
(b. 1938), haemato-oncologist:
Leukaemia.

Dr Ann Prentice
(b. 1952), nutritionist:
Breastfeeding.

Professor Colin Prentice
(1934–2014), physician:
Platelets.

Professor Laurie Prescott
(b. 1934), clinical pharmacologist:
Clinical Pharmacology 1.

Dr Elizabeth Price
(b. 1944), medical microbiologist:
MRSA.

Professor Brian Prichard
(1932–2010), Secretary of the British
Pharmacological Society:
*Clinical Pharmacology 1, Clinical
Pharmacology 2.*

Professor Kalevi Pyörälä
(b. 1930), physician:
Cholesterol.

Mrs Vicky Quarshie
(b. 1972), Headache Nurse Specialist:
Migraine.

Dr Rosaline Quinlivan
(b. 1959), Paediatrician:
Muscular Dystrophy.

Professor Tom Quinn
(b. 1961), professor of cardiovascular
nursing:
Platelets.

Professor Pat Rabbitt
(b. 1934), psychologist:
Applied Psychology.

Professor Maja Račić
(b. 1972), family practitioner:
Rural Medicine.

Sir George Radda
(b. 1936), radiologist, former President
of the Society for Magnetic Resonance
in Medicine:
NMR and MRI.

Professor Sandy Raeburn
(b. 1941), clinical geneticist, and former
Chairman of the Scottish Council of
the Cystic Fibrosis Research Trust:
Cystic Fibrosis.

Mrs Jennifer Raiman
(b. 1936), developer of London
Hospital Pain Chart:
Pain.

Ms Jane Randall-Smith
(b. 1953), medical administrator:
Rural Medicine.

Professor Chris Rawlings
(b. 1954), bioinformatician:
Gene Mapping, Individual Interview.

Professor Sir Michael Rawlins
(b. 1941), clinical pharmacologist,
member of National Committee on
Pharmacology and Committee on
Safety of Medicines:
Clinical Pharmacology 2.

Professor Andrew Read
(b. 1939), medical geneticist:
Clinical Molecular Genetics.

Mr John Read
orthopaedic surgeon:
Hip Replacement.

Dr Malcolm Read
(b. 1941), medical officer to
Commonwealth and Olympic Games:
Sports Medicine.

Mr Howard Rees
(b. 1928), veterinary officer:
Foot and Mouth.

Dame Lesley Rees
(b. 1942), chemical endocrinologist:
Endogenous Opiates.

Professor John Reid
(b. 1943), clinical pharmacologist:
*Clinical Pharmacology 1, Clinical
Pharmacology 2.*

Professor Mary Renfrew
(b. 1955), professor of midwifery:
Breastfeeding.

Mrs Brenda Reynolds
mother of paediatric oncology patient:
Platinum Salts.

Professor Gavin Reynolds
(b. 1952), neuroscientist:
5-HT, Brain Banks.

Mrs Lois Reynolds
(b. 1947) medical historian:
Applied Psychology.

Professor Osmund Reynolds
(b. 1933), perinatal and neonatal
paediatrician:
Neonatal Intensive Care, NMR and MRI.

Professor Graham Richards
(b. 1941), historian of psychology:
Applied Psychology.

Professor Martin Richards
(b. 1940), professor of family research:
Ethics of Genetics.

Professor Sir Rex Richards
(b. 1922), chemist:
NMR and MRI.

Dr Alan Richardson
(b. 1940), veterinary surgeon:
Foot and Mouth.

Professor Peter Richardson
(b. 1935), engineer:
Platelets.

Professor Sir Mark Richmond
(b. 1931), biochemist, microbiologist:
MRSA.

Dr Sam Richmond
(b. 1949), neonatologist:
Corticosteroids.

Professor Povl Riis
(1925–2017), former Chairman of
the Danish National Sciences Ethical
Committee:
Medical Ethics.

Dr Julia Riley
(b. 1960), palliative care specialist:
Palliative Medicine.

Mr Peter Ring
(b. 1922), orthopaedic surgeon:
Hip Replacement.

Dr Sue Ring
(b. 1967), geneticist:
ALSPAC.

Professor Jim Ritter
(b. 1944), clinical pharmacologist:
Clinical Pharmacology 1.

Dr Rodney Rivers
(b. 1939), neonatologist:
Neonatal Intensive Care.

Dr Geoffrey Rivett
(b. 1932), Department of Health and
medical historian:
Heart Transplant, Public Health.

Dr Charles Rizza
(b. 1930), consultant physician:
Haemophilia.

Professor Derek Roberts
(b. 1925), geneticist:
Genetic Testing.

Dr Angela Robinson
(b. 1942), paediatric haematologist:
Rhesus Factor.

Professor Jean Robinson
Honorary Research Officer for the
Association for Improvements in the
Maternity Services (UK):
Maternal Care, Ultrasound.

Dr Philip Robson
(b. 1947), clinical and industrial
pharmacologist, psychiatrist:
Cannabis.

Professor Charles Rodeck
(b. 1944), clinician, researcher in foetal
medicine:
Genetic Testing, Rhesus Factor.

Dr Keith Rogers
(1910–2005), consultant
microbiologist:
Post Penicillin.

Dr Peter Rohde
(b. 1933), psychiatrist:
Psychiatric Drugs.

Professor Ivan Roitt
(b. 1927), immunologist:
Autoimmunity.

Dr Stanley Rosen
nephrologist:
Dialysis.

Professor Norman Rosenthal
(b. 1950), psychiatrist:
SAD, Individual Interview.

Mr Barry Ross
(b. 1934), thoracic surgeon:
Heart Transplant.

Mr Donald Ross
(1922–2014), consultant cardiac
surgeon:
Heart Transplant.

Sir Keith Ross
(1927–2003), consultant cardiac
surgeon:
Heart Transplant.

Professor James Rourke
(b. 1952), rural GP and medical
educator:
Rural Medicine.

Professor Phil Routledge
(b. 1948), clinical pharmacologist:
*Clinical Pharmacology 1, Clinical
Pharmacology 2.*

Professor David Rowlands
(b. 1940), veterinary virologist:
Foot and Mouth.

Dr John Rudd
(b. 1967), physiologist:
Platinum Salts.

Dame Joan Ruddock
(b. 1943), Member of Parliament:
Waste, Individual Interview.

Mrs Patti Rundall
(b. 1950), baby food campaigner:
Breastfeeding.

Dr George Russell
(b. 1936), paediatrician:
Asthma.

Dr Ethan Russo
(b. 1952), pharmaceutical scientist/
industrial adviser:
Cannabis.

Professor Sir Michael Rutter
(b. 1933), child and adolescent
psychiatrist:
Individual Interview.

Mrs Sue Sadler
(b. 1943), clinic manager at ALSPAC:
ALSPAC.

Dr Stewart Sage
(b. 1962), physiologist:
Platelets.

Professor Jeremy Saklatvala
(b. 1943), rheumatologist:
TNF.

Ms Ellena Salariya
(b. 1931), midwife/breastfeeding
educator and researcher:
Breastfeeding.

Professor Julian Sampson
(b. 1959), medical geneticist:
*Clinical Cancer Genetics, Clinical
Molecular Genetics.*

Professor Thomas Sanders
(b. 1949), professor of nutrition:
Cholesterol.

Professor Merton Sandler
(1926–2014), pharmacologist:
5-HT, Migraine, Psychiatric Drugs.

Professor Gareth Sanger
(b. 1953), pharmacologist:
5-HT, Platinum Salts, Individual Interview.

Professor Peter Sasieni
(b. 1963), biostatistician:
Cervical Cancer.

Dame Cicely Saunders
(1918–2005), physician, founder of
modern hospice movement:
Pain.

Professor Wendy Savage
(b. 1935), obstetrician and
gynaecologist:
Maternal Care.

Dr Felicity Savage
(b. 1939), community paediatrician:
Breastfeeding.

Mr John Sawkins
(b. 1946), lab technician:
NIMR, Individual Interview.

Professor Pramod Saxena
(b. 1939), pharmacologist:
Migraine.

Professor Guy Scadding
(1907–1999), professor of medicine:
Clinical Research.

Mr Chris Schermbrucker
(b. 1935), veterinary vaccinologist:
Foot and Mouth.

Dr Donald Scott
(b. 1930), clinical neurophysiologist:
Psychiatric Drugs.

Dr Geoffrey Scott
(b. 1948), clinical microbiologist:
MRSA, Post Penicillin, TB Chemotherapy.

Professor James Scott
(1924–2006), obstetrician and
gynaecologist:
Rhesus Factor.

Professor James Scott
(b. 1946), consultant physician:
Cholesterol.

Dr Jo Scott-Jones
(b. 1963), rural GP:
Rural Medicine.

Professor Clive Seale
(b. 1955), medical sociologist:
NATSAL, Palliative Medicine.

Professor Anthony Seaton
(b. 1938), respiratory and occupational
health physician:
Air Pollution, Individual Interview.

Dr David Secher
immunologist and technology transfer
specialist:
Monoclonal Antibodies.

Dr Joseph Selkon
(1928–2013), consultant
microbiologist:
MRSA.

Dr Bob Sellers
(b. 1924), veterinary virologist:
Foot and Mouth.

Miss Mary Selsby
(b. 1934), renal nurse, dialysis services
manager:
Dialysis.

Professor Jane Seymour
(b. 1958), palliative care nurse:
Palliative Medicine.

Professor Stanley Shaldon
(1931–2013), nephrologist, home dialysis pioneer:
Dialysis.

Dr Rosemary Shannon
(b. 1943), consultant paediatric oncologist:
Leukaemia.

Dr David Shanson
(b. 1944), medical microbiologist:
MRSA.

Professor Gerry Shaper
(b. 1927), clinical epidemiologist:
Africa, Cholesterol.

Mr Ernie Sharp
(1921–2015), waste manager:
Waste, Individual Interview.

Ms Karen Shaw
(b. 1964), research/brain donation nurse:
Brain Banks.

Dr Julian Shelley
(b. 1932), pharmacologist:
Clinical Pharmacology 2.

Professor Roger Short
(b. 1930), reproductive biologist:
Breastfeeding.

The Very Revd Edward Shotter
(b. 1933), medical ethicist:
Medical Ethics.

Dr Ann Silver
(b. 1929), physiologist:
Individual Interview.

Dr John Silver
(b. 1931), spinal injuries specialist:
Rhesus Factor.

Professor Michael Silverman
(b. 1943), paediatrician:
Asthma.

Dr Norman Simmons
(b. 1933), medical microbiologist:
MRSA.

Dr Dennis Simms
(b. 1926), civil servant:
Environmental Toxicology.

Professor Albert Singer
(b. 1938), obstetrician/gynaecologist:
Cervical Cancer.

Professor Mervyn Singer
(b. 1958), physician, intensive care consultant:
Intensive Care.

Sir John Skehel
(b. 1941), virologist:
Common Cold Unit.

Dr Rosalind Skinner
(b. 1946), clinical geneticist:
Clinical Molecular Genetics.

Professor Heather Skirton
(b. 1953), nurse consultant, genetic counsellor:
Clinical Genetics.

Dr Norman Slark
(b. 1934), physicist and medical civil servant:
Ultrasound.

Dr Brian Slawson
(b. 1933), consultant anaesthetist:
Intensive Care.

Dr Mary Smale
(b. 1943), breastfeeding counsellor:
Breastfeeding.

Professor Rod Smallwood
(b. 1945), medical engineer:
Medical Physics.

Dr Jean Smellie
(b. 1927), paediatrician:
Neonatal Intensive Care, Rhesus Factor.

Dr Alec Smith
(1927–2014), tropical medicine
expert:
Africa.

Professor Alwyn Smith
(1925–2016), epidemiologist:
Public Health.

Professor Dale Smith
(b. 1951), medical historian:
MRSA.

Dr Elspeth Smith
(b. 1923), biochemist:
Cholesterol.

Dr Jim Smith
(b. 1954), molecular developmental
biologist:
NIMR.

Dr John Smith
(b. 1953), histopathologist:
Cervical Cancer.

Dr Lindsay Smith
(b. 1957), GP:
Maternal Care.

Professor Robert Smith
toxicologist:
Environmental Toxicology.

Dr Robert (Bob) N Smith
(b. 1934), pharmaceutical medical
director:
Clinical Pharmacology 2.

Dr Roger Smith
(b. 1945), cardiologist:
Platelets.

Dr Derek Smyth
(b. 1927), biochemist:
Endogenous Opiates.

Dr Bob Snow
(b. 1961), epidemiologist:
Africa.

Professor Ellen Solomon
(b. 1943), human geneticist:
Clinical Cancer Genetics, Gene Mapping.

Dr Jane Somerville
(b. 1933), cardiologist:
Heart Transplant.

Dr Walter Somerville
(1913–2005), cardiologist:
Heart Transplant.

Dr Pam Sonnenberg
(b. 1965), infectious disease
epidemiologist:
NATSAL.

Lord Soulsby
(b. 1926), veterinary surgeon and
trade unionist:
Foot and Mouth.

Professor Anne Soutar
(b. 1945), biochemist:
Cholesterol.

Dr Kevin Southern
(b. 1964), paediatrician:
Cystic Fibrosis.

Dr Geoffrey Spencer
(b. 1929), consultant anaesthetist:
Intensive Care.

Dr Ian Spencer
(b. 1961), medical historian:
Ultrasound.

Professor Peter Sperryn
(b. 1937), sports medicine consultant:
Sports Medicine.

Professor Maura Spiegel
(b. 1954), narrative medicine scholar:
Narrative Medicine.

Dr Alison Spiro
(b. 1949), health visitor/breastfeeding
counsellor:
Breastfeeding.

Professor Brian Spratt
(b. 1947), molecular microbiologist:
MRSA.

Dr Arthur Spriggs
(1919–2015), cytopathologist:
Cervical Cancer.

Dr Bertie Squire
(b. 1960), infectious diseases expert:
TB Chemotherapy.

Dr Anthony Selwyn St Leger
(b. 1948), epidemiologist:
*Population-based Research, Individual
Interview.*

Dr David Stableforth
(b. 1942), consultant physician in adult
cystic fibrosis care:
Cystic Fibrosis.

Professor Margaret Stanley
(b. 1939), cytopathologist:
Cervical Cancer.

Professor Stephen Stansfeld
(b. 1951), psychiatrist:
Population-based Research.

Dr Penny Stanway
(b. 1946), GP:
Breastfeeding.

Professor Hannah Steinberg
(b. 1924), psychopharmacologist:
Endogenous Opiates, Psychiatric Drugs.

Professor Robert Steiner
(1918–2013), radiologist:
NMR and MRI, Peptic Ulcer.

Mr Ian Stephen
(b. 1944), orthopaedic surgeon:
Hip Replacement.

Professor Andrew Stevens
(b. 1954), professor of public health:
Platelets.

Dr Ann Stewart
(1930–2004), paediatrician:
Neonatal Intensive Care.

Professor Gordon Stewart
(b. 1919), public health physician:
MRSA, Post Penicillin.

Professor Gordon Stirrat
(b. 1940), obstetrician and
gynaecologist:
ALSPAC.

Professor Jan Stjernswärd
(b. 1936), palliative care specialist:
Pain.

Dr John Stock
(b. 1919), chemist/pharmacologist:
Leukaemia.

Dame Barbara Stocking
(b. 1951), charity chief executive
and early recipient of corticosteroid
therapy:
Corticosteroids.

Dr Joseph Stoddart
(b. 1932), consultant anaesthetist:
Intensive Care.

Professor David Strachan
(b. 1957), epidemiologist:
Population-based Research.

Professor Roger Strasser
(b. 1952), rural physician and medical
educator:
Rural Medicine.

Professor Sarah Strasser
(b. 1955), rural physician and medical
educator:
Rural Medicine.

Professor Leo Strunin
(b. 1937), anaesthetist:
Intensive Care.

Ms Fiona Stuart
(b. 1955), MAFF veterinary officer:
Bovine TB.

Professor Steve Sturdy
(b. 1957), medical sociologist and
historian:
Muscular Dystrophy.

Dr Maurice Super
(1936–2006), consultant paediatric
geneticist:
Cystic Fibrosis.

Professor Ian Sutherland
(b. 1945), biomedical engineer:
NIMR.

Dr Robert Sutherland
(b. 1930), bacteriologist:
MRSA.

Mr Malcolm Swann
(b. 1931), orthopaedic surgeon for
juvenile chronic arthritis:
Hip Replacement.

Professor Alan Swanson
(b. 1931), professor of biomechanics:
Hip Replacement.

Mr Peter Sweetnam
(b. 1941), medical statistician:
*Population-based Research, Individual
Interview.*

Sir Rodney Sweetnam
(1927–2013), orthopaedic surgeon:
Hip Replacement.

Dr Mark Swerdlow
(1918–2003), consultant anaesthetist:
Pain.

Professor Cameron Swift
(b. 1946), clinical pharmacologist:
Clinical Pharmacology 2.

Professor Elizabeth Sykes
(b. 1936), psychopharmacologist:
Psychiatric Drugs.

Professor Sir Keith Sykes
(b. 1925), consultant anaesthetist:
Intensive Care.

Mrs Marilyn Symonds
(b. 1947), cytologist:
Cervical Cancer.

Dr Anne Szarewski
(1959–2013), epidemiologist:
Cervical Cancer.

Dr Ian Tait
(1926–2013), GP and medical
historian:
*General Practice, Maternal Care, Medical
Ethics, Psychiatric Drugs.*

Professor Ann Taket
(b. 1954), primary healthcare specialist:
Public Health.

The Revd Alan Tanner
(1925–2015), chairman of the
Haemophilia Society:
Haemophilia.

Professor Tilli Tansey
(b. 1953), neuroscientist, historian of
modern medical sciences:
*5-HT, Air Pollution, Africa, ALSPAC,
Applied Psychology, Brain Banks,
Breastfeeding, Cannabis, Cervical
Cancer, Clinical Cancer Genetics, Clinical
Genetics, Clinical Molecular Genetics,
Clinical Pharmacology 1, Clinical
Pharmacology 2, Common Cold Unit,
Corticosteroids, Dialysis, Endogenous
Opiates, Ethics of Genetics, Gene
Mapping, Foot and Mouth, Haemophilia,
Intensive Care, Intestinal Absorption,
Leukaemia, Maternal Care, Medical
Ethics, Migraine, Muscular Dystrophy,
Narrative Medicine, NATSAL, Neonatal
Intensive Care, NIMR, Palliative Medicine,
Peptic Ulcer, Platelets, Platinum Salts,
Post Penicillin, Psychiatric Drugs,
Rural Medicine, SAD, Safety of Drugs,
Sports Medicine, TNF, Tobacco Control,
Ultrasound, Waste.*

Dr David Tattersall
(b. 1961), neuropharmacologist:
Platinum Salts.

Professor Peter Tavner
(b. 1946), engineer:
Air Pollution.

Mr Angus Taylor
(b. 1917), veterinary surgeon:
Foot and Mouth.

Dr Suzanne Taylor
(b. 1978), medical historian:
Cannabis.

Professor Karen Temple
clinical geneticist:
Muscular Dystrophy.

Dr Adrian Thomas
(b. 1954), radiologist:
Medical Physics.

Dr Duncan Thomas
(b. 1929), haematologist:
Platelets.

Dr Hugh Thomas
(b. 1952), GP:
*Common Cold Unit, Population-based
Research.*

**Ms Mary Thomas
(Mrs Hart)**
(b. 1940), epidemiology field worker:
Population-based Research.

Mrs Wendy Thomas
(b. 1949), Chief Executive of the
Migraine Trust:
Migraine.

Mr Mark Thomasin-Foster
(b. 1943), farmer and environmentalist:
Bovine TB.

Professor Harry Thomason
(b. 1940), sports scientist:
Sports Medicine.

Professor Gilbert Thompson
(b. 1932), physician:
Cholesterol.

Mr Keith Thompson
(b. 1926), medical administrator:
Common Cold Unit.

Professor Andrew Thomson
(b. 1940), chemist:
Platinum Salts.

Mr Paul Thornber
(b. 1945), waste management
executive:
Waste.

Mrs Vicky Tinsley
(b. 1960), midwife and manager:
Maternal Care.

Dr Patricia Tippett
(b. 1930), haematology research
worker:
Genetic Testing, Rhesus Factor.

Dr Jonathan Tobert
(b. 1945), pharmaceutical physician:
Cholesterol.

Dr Paul Tofts
(b. 1949), medical physicist:
NMR and MRI.

Dr Peter Tothill
(b. 1922), medical physicist:
Medical Physics.

Dr Derrick Tovey
(b. 1926), transfusion centre director:
Rhesus Factor.

Mr Frank Tovey
(b. 1921), surgeon:
Peptic Ulcer.

Professor Anthony Travis
(b. 1943), historian of chemistry:
NIMR.

Professor Tom Treasure
(b. 1947), cardiothoracic surgeon:
Heart Transplant, NMR and MRI.

Professor Geoffrey Tucker
(b. 1943), pharmacologist:
Clinical Pharmacology 1.

Mr Keith Tucker
(b. 1945), orthopaedic surgeon,
founder member of the British Hip
Society:
Hip Replacement.

Professor Edward Tuddenham
(b. 1944), haematologist:
Haemophilia.

Mr Theodore Tulley
(b. 1918), physicist:
Medical Physics.

Dr Dan Tunstall Pedoe
(1939–2015), consultant cardiologist:
Sports Medicine.

Professor Hugh Tunstall-Pedoe
(b. 1939), cardiovascular
epidemiologist:
Cholesterol.

Lord (Leslie) Turnberg
(b. 1934), gastroenterologist/
physiologist:
Intestinal Absorption.

Professor Neil Turner
(b. 1956), nephrologist:
Dialysis.

Mr Peter Turner
(b. 1949), head technician, parasitology:
NIMR.

Dr Trevor Turner
(b. 1948), psychiatrist:
Psychiatric Drugs.

Mr Wilfred Turner
former diplomat, Secretary to the
Committee on Safety of Drugs from
1963 to 1966:
Safety of Drugs.

Dr John Turney
(b. 1948), consultant renal physician:
Dialysis.

Professor Peter Turnpenny
(b. 1953), clinical geneticist:
Ethics of Genetics.

Dr Robert Twycross
(b. 1941), clinician and researcher in
palliative medicine:
Pain, Palliative Medicine.

Dr Mike Tyers
(b. 1946), industrial pharmacologist:
5-HT.

Dr Linda Tyfield
(b. 1946), molecular geneticist:
ALSPAC.

Dr David Tyrrell
(1925–2005), medical virologist:
*Africa, Applied Psychology, Autoimmunity,
Clinical Research, Common Cold Unit,
Endogenous Opiates, General Practice,
Genetic Testing, Haemophilia, Heart
Transplant, Monoclonal Antibodies, Peptic
Ulcer, Population-based Research, Post
Penicillin.*

Mr Ken Tyrrell
(1929–2001), veterinary surgeon:
Foot and Mouth.

Professor Timos Valaes
(b. 1927), neonatologist:
Rhesus Factor.

Professor Sir Patrick Vallance
(b. 1960), pharmacologist:
Clinical Pharmacology 1.

Professor Veronica van Heyningen
(b. 1946), molecular geneticist:
Gene Mapping.

Professor Gert-Jan van Ommen
(b.1947), geneticist:
Muscular Dystrophy.

Professor Duncan Vere
(b. 1929), clinical pharmacologist:
*Clinical Pharmacology 1, Clinical
Pharmacology 2, Pain.*

The Revd Bryan Vernon
(b. 1950), ethicist:
Medical Ethics.

Dr Roger Verrier Jones
(b. 1934), paediatrician:
Corticosteroids.

Dr Marcos Vidal
(1974–2016), cancer biologist:
TNF.

Dr Glyn Volans
(b. 1943), pharmacologist:
Migraine.

Professor Keir Waddington
(b. 1970), medical historian:
Bovine TB.

Professor Owen Wade
(1921–2008), physician, clinical
pharmacologist:
*Clinical Pharmacology 1, Clinical
Pharmacology 2, Population-based
Research, Safety of Drugs.*

Dr Milton Wainwright
(b. 1950), microbiologist:
Post Penicillin.

Professor Henning Walczak
(b. 1966), cancer researcher:
TNF.

Professor Leslie Walker
(b. 1949), social pyschologist:
Cervical Cancer.

Mr Patrick Walker
(b. 1949), Consultant gynaecologist:
Cervical Cancer.

Professor John Walker-Smith
(b. 1936), paediatric gastroenterologist:
Cystic Fibrosis, Intestinal Absorption, Leukaemia, Pain.

Mr Mike Wall
(b. 1965), ALSPAC parent:
ALSPAC.

Professor Patrick Wall
(1925–2001), physiologist:
Pain.

Dr Susan Wallace
(b. 1960), geneticist, medical administrator:
Gene Mapping.

Professor David Wallis
(b. 1934), pharmacologist:
5-HT.

Professor John Wallwork
(b. 1946), transplant surgeon:
Heart Transplant.

Sir Mark Walport
(b. 1953), UK Government Chief Scientific Adviser, former Director of the Wellcome Trust (2003–2013):
Clinical Pharmacology 1.

Professor Dafydd Walters
(b. 1947), paediatrician:
Air Pollution, Corticosteroids.

Dr Heather Walton
(b. 1962), environmental health researcher:
Air Pollution.

Lord (John) Walton
(1922–2016), neurologist:
Clinical Research.

Mr Humphry Ward
(b. 1938), obstetrician and gynaecologist:
Rhesus Factor.

Dr Jill Warner
(b. 1962), allergist:
Asthma.

Professor John Warner
(b. 1945), paediatrician:
Asthma.

Mrs Jenny Warren
(b. 1946), former National Breastfeeding Adviser for Scotland:
Breastfeeding.

Professor Elizabeth Warrington
(b. 1931), neuropsychologist:
Individual Interview.

John Waterlow
(1916–2010), nutritionist:
Africa.

Professor Estlin Waters
(b. 1934), epidemiologist:
Population-based Research, Individual Interview.

Miss Pamela Waterworth
(1920–2004), microbiologist:
Post Penicillin.

Professor Sir David Weatherall
(b. 1933), molecular geneticist:
Clinical Genetics, Clinical Molecular Genetics, Genetic Testing, Leukaemia, Rhesus Factor.

Dr Josephine Weatherall
medical statistician:
Safety of Drugs.

Dr Mark Weatherall
(b. 1968), consultant neurologist:
Migraine.

Professor Miles Weatherall
(1920–2007), pharmacologist:
Common Cold Unit, Endogenous Opiates, Monoclonal Antibodies, Safety of Drugs.

Professor Lawrence Weaver
(b. 1948), paediatrician:
Breastfeeding.

Professor David Webb
(b. 1953), clinical pharmacologist:
Clinical Pharmacology 1.

Professor Kevin Webb
(b. 1946), clinician in cystic fibrosis adult care:
Cystic Fibrosis.

Dr Jean Weddell
(1928–2013), scientific staff member of the MRC Epidemiology Research Unit:
Population-based Research.

Professor Bee Wee
(b. 1964), palliative care specialist:
Palliative Medicine.

Professor Joanna Weinberg,
psychiatrist:
Psychiatric Drugs.

Mr Clifford Welch
(b. 1925), former Chairman of the Katharine Dormandy Trust:
Haemophilia.

Professor Kaye Wellings
(b. 1948), co–founder of NATSAL:
NATSAL.

Mr John Wells
(b. 1944), industrial nutritionist:
Breastfeeding.

Professor Peter Wells
(b. 1936), medical physicist:
Medical Physics, Ultrasound.

Professor John West
(b. 1928), physiologist:
Applied Psychology, Medical Physics, MRSA.

Professor Brian Wharton
(b. 1937), professor of human nutrition:
Breastfeeding.

Dr David Wheatley
(b. 1929), consultant psychiatrist:
Psychiatric Drugs.

Mr Victor Wheble
(b. 1919), orthopaedic surgeon:
Hip Replacement.

Dame Margaret Wheeler
(b. 1932), midwife:
Maternal Care.

Mr Steven White
(b. 1955), engineer:
NIMR.

Professor Roger Whitehead
(b. 1933), director of child nutrition research:
Africa, Breastfeeding.

Professor Charles Whitfield
(b. 1927), consultant obstetrician:
*Maternal Care, Rhesus Factor,
Ultrasound.*

Dr Tony Whittingham
(b. 1944), medical physicist:
Ultrasound.

Professor John Widdicombe
(1925–2011), physiologist:
Cystic Fibrosis.

Professor Jonathan Wigglesworth
(b. 1932), perinatal pathologist:
Neonatal Intensive Care.

Mr Tony Wilkes
(b. 1933), entomologist:
Africa.

Mr Adam Wilkinson
(b. 1977), administrator:
Bovine TB.

Mr John Wilkinson
(b. 1944), physicist:
Medical Physics.

Dr Lise Wilkinson
medical virologist, medical historian:
Foot and Mouth.

Dr Peter Wilkinson
(b. 1945), medical microbiologist:
Medical Ethics.

Dr Michael Wilks
forensic medical examiner:
Medical Ethics.

Dr Eric (Es) Will
(b. 1945), nephrologist,
bioinformatician:
Individual Interview

Dr Anthony Williams
(b. 1951), paediatrician:
Breastfeeding.

Miss Carol Williams
public health nutritionist:
Breastfeeding.

Mr David Williams
(1940–2013), Chair of the Badger
Trust:
Bovine TB.

Sir David Innes Williams
(1919–2013), urological surgeon:
Clinical Research.

Mr John Williams
(b. 1945), obstetrician and
gynaecologist:
Corticosteroids.

Professor Martin Williams
(b. 1947), environmental chemist:
Air Pollution.

Dr Peter Williams
(1925–2014), medical administrator,
Director of the Wellcome Trust
(1965–1991):
*Africa, Clinical Research, Common Cold
Unit, Intestinal Absorption, Monoclonal
Antibodies, NATSAL.*

Professor Peter Williams
(b. 1949), medical physicist:
Medical Physics.

Professor Richard Williams
(b. 1956), immunologist:
TNF.

Professor Robert Williams
(1926–2015), inorganic chemist:
Platinum Salts.

Mrs Sally Williams
(b. 1936), physiotherapist:
Sports Medicine.

Mrs Wendy Williams
(b. 1941), survey interviewer:
NATSAL.

Dr W O Williams
(b. 1921), GP:
General Practice.

Professor Robert (Bob) Williamson
(b. 1938), geneticist:
Clinical Molecular Genetics.

Dr James Willocks
(b. 1928), obstetrician:
Ultrasound.

Professor David Wilson
(b. 1952), environmental chemist:
Waste.

Mr Michael Wilson
(b. 1956), orthopaedic surgeon:
Hip Replacement.

Dr Eve Wiltshaw
(b. 1927), oncologist:
Leukaemia, Platinum Salts.

Dr Guil Winchester
medical historian:
Monoclonal Antibodies.

Professor Jan Witkowski
(b. 1947), molecular biologist and
medical historian:
Muscular Dystrophy.

Dr Margaret Wolfendale
(b. 1931), cytopathologist:
Cervical Cancer.

Professor Heinz Wolff
(b. 1928), bioengineer and television
presenter:
NIMR.

Dr John Wood
(b. 1949), pharmacologist:
Peptic Ulcer.

Professor Sir Martin Wood
(b. 1927), medical technology
developer in industry:
NMR and MRI.

Professor Ciaran Woodman
(1954–2015), cancer epidemiologist:
Cervical Cancer.

Professor John Woodrow
(b. 1924), consultant physician:
Genetic Testing, Rhesus Factor.

Professor Abigail Woods
(b. 1972), medical historian:
Foot and Mouth.

Professor Frank Woods
(1937–2016), pharmacologist:
*Clinical Pharmacology 1, Environmental
Toxicology.*

Dr James (Jim) Woody
pharmaceutical development specialist:
TNF.

Professor Neville Woolf
(b. 1930), histopathologist:
Cholesterol.

Dr Michael Woolridge
(b. 1950), infant nutrition researcher:
Breastfeeding.

Professor Brian Worthington
(1938–2007), radiologist:
NMR and MRI.

Dr David Wright
(b. 1944), anaesthetist:
Intensive Care.

Dr Martin Wright
(1912–2001), bioengineer:
Population-based Research.

Mr Mick Wright
(b. 1949), waste manager:
Waste, Individual Interview.

Mrs Sheila Wright
(b. 1919), MRC publications officer:
Population-based Research.

Professor B Michael Wroblewski
(b. 1934), orthopaedic surgeon:
Hip Replacement.

Professor Oliver Wrong
(1925–2012), nephrologist:
Intestinal Absorption.

Professor John Wyatt
(b. 1952), neonatologist:
Neonatal Intensive Care.

Dr John Wynn-Jones
(b. 1951), rural GP:
Rural Medicine.

Dr John Yarnell
epidemiologist:
Population-based Research, Individual Interview.

Professor John Yates
(b. 1948), medical geneticist:
Clinical Molecular Genetics.

Dr Alan Yoshioka
(b. 1963), medical historian:
Post Penicillin.

Mrs Elisabeth Young
(b. 1942), biochemist in paediatric pathology:
Genetic Testing.

Professor Ian Young
(b. 1932), physicist:
NMR and MRI.

Professor Maureen Young
(1915–2013), perinatal physiologist:
Neonatal Intensive Care.

Professor John S Yudkin
(b. 1943), professor of nutrition:
Cholesterol.

Professor Doris Zallen
(b. 1941), medical historian:
Genetic Testing, Rhesus Factor.

Dr Luke Zander
(b. 1935), GP:
Maternal Care.

Dr Thomas Zeltner
(b. 1947), public health specialist and WHO adviser:
Tobacco Control.

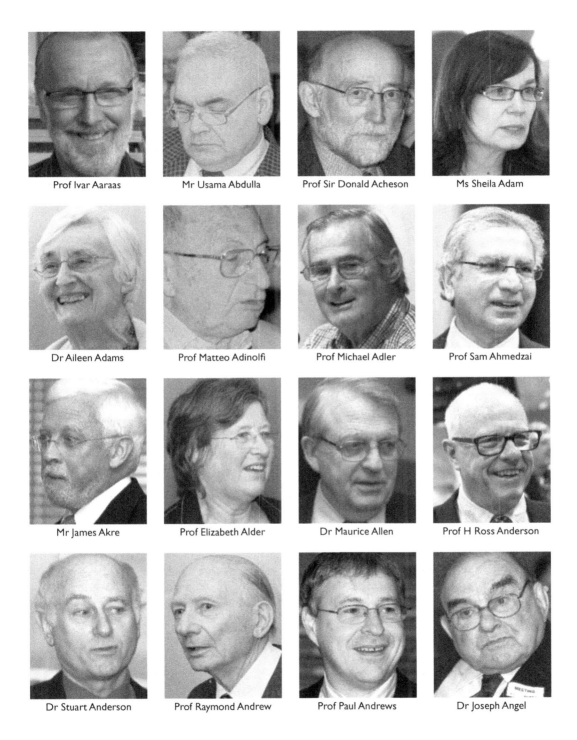

Prof Ivar Aaraas	Mr Usama Abdulla	Prof Sir Donald Acheson	Ms Sheila Adam
Dr Aileen Adams	Prof Matteo Adinolfi	Prof Michael Adler	Prof Sam Ahmedzai
Mr James Akre	Prof Elizabeth Alder	Dr Maurice Allen	Prof H Ross Anderson
Dr Stuart Anderson	Prof Raymond Andrew	Prof Paul Andrews	Dr Joseph Angel

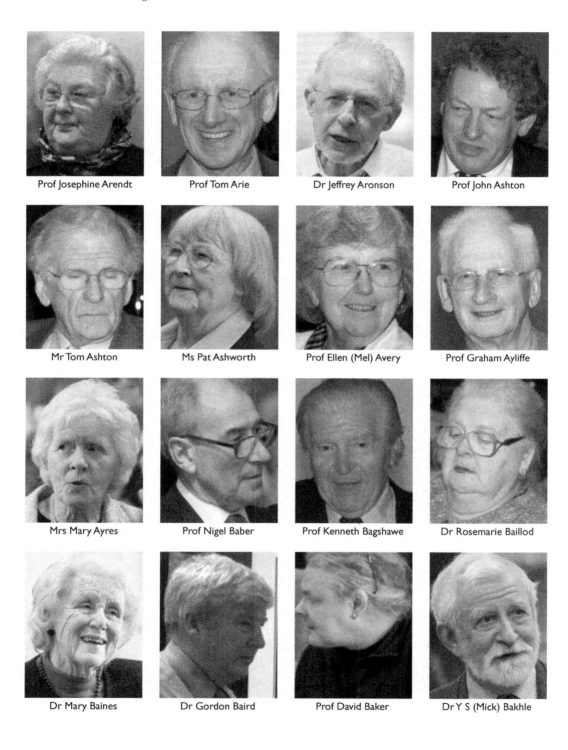

Prof Josephine Arendt

Prof Tom Arie

Dr Jeffrey Aronson

Prof John Ashton

Mr Tom Ashton

Ms Pat Ashworth

Prof Ellen (Mel) Avery

Prof Graham Ayliffe

Mrs Mary Ayres

Prof Nigel Baber

Prof Kenneth Bagshawe

Dr Rosemarie Baillod

Dr Mary Baines

Dr Gordon Baird

Prof David Baker

Dr Y S (Mick) Bakhle

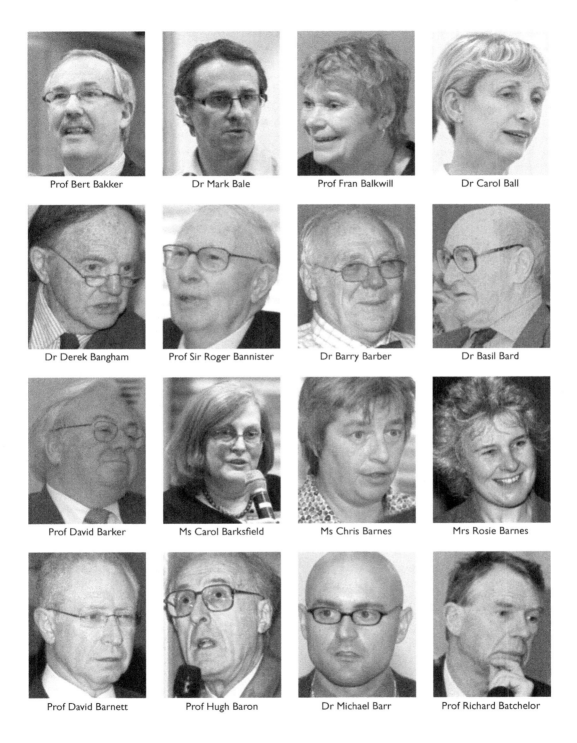

Prof Bert Bakker   Dr Mark Bale   Prof Fran Balkwill   Dr Carol Ball

Dr Derek Bangham   Prof Sir Roger Bannister   Dr Barry Barber   Dr Basil Bard

Prof David Barker   Ms Carol Barksfield   Ms Chris Barnes   Mrs Rosie Barnes

Prof David Barnett   Prof Hugh Baron   Dr Michael Barr   Prof Richard Batchelor

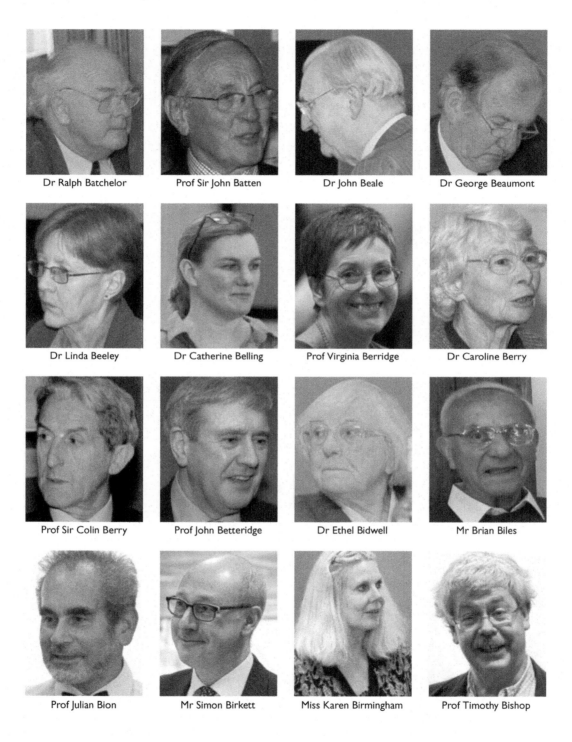

Dr Ralph Batchelor

Prof Sir John Batten

Dr John Beale

Dr George Beaumont

Dr Linda Beeley

Dr Catherine Belling

Prof Virginia Berridge

Dr Caroline Berry

Prof Sir Colin Berry

Prof John Betteridge

Dr Ethel Bidwell

Mr Brian Biles

Prof Julian Bion

Mr Simon Birkett

Miss Karen Birmingham

Prof Timothy Bishop

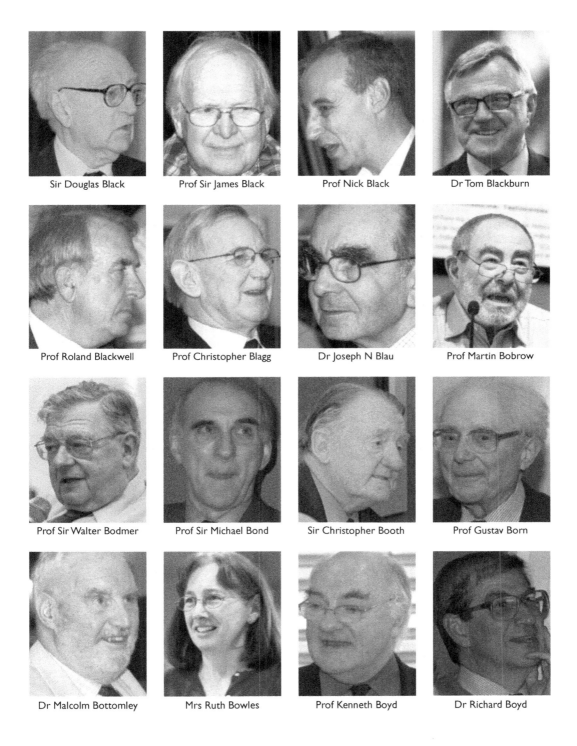

Sir Douglas Black

Prof Sir James Black

Prof Nick Black

Dr Tom Blackburn

Prof Roland Blackwell

Prof Christopher Blagg

Dr Joseph N Blau

Prof Martin Bobrow

Prof Sir Walter Bodmer

Prof Sir Michael Bond

Sir Christopher Booth

Prof Gustav Born

Dr Malcolm Bottomley

Mrs Ruth Bowles

Prof Kenneth Boyd

Dr Richard Boyd

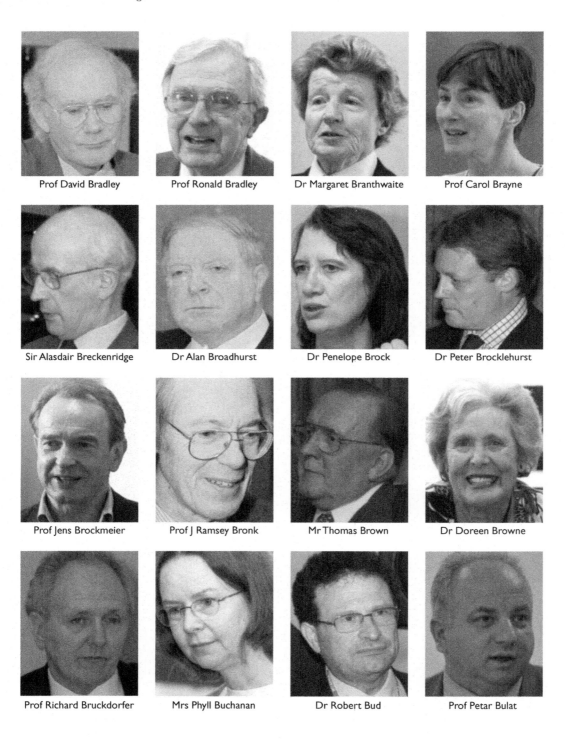

Prof David Bradley

Prof Ronald Bradley

Dr Margaret Branthwaite

Prof Carol Brayne

Sir Alasdair Breckenridge

Dr Alan Broadhurst

Dr Penelope Brock

Dr Peter Brocklehurst

Prof Jens Brockmeier

Prof J Ramsey Bronk

Mr Thomas Brown

Dr Doreen Browne

Prof Richard Bruckdorfer

Mrs Phyll Buchanan

Dr Robert Bud

Prof Petar Bulat

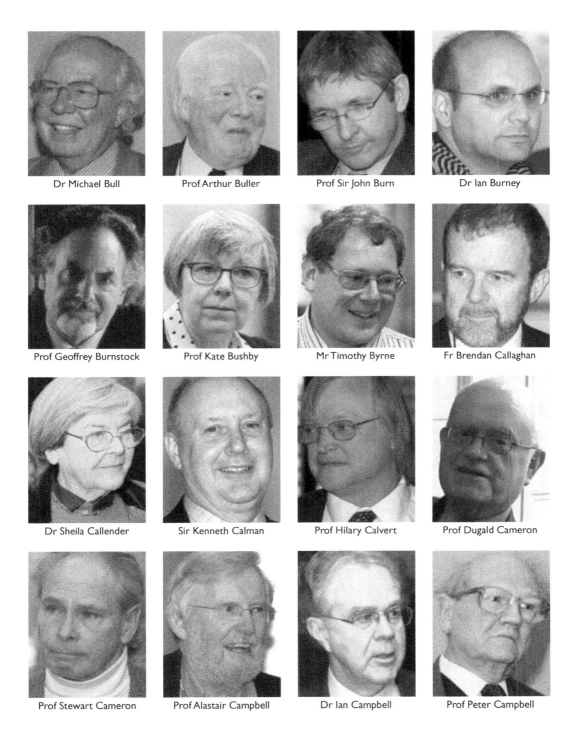

Dr Michael Bull Prof Arthur Buller Prof Sir John Burn Dr Ian Burney

Prof Geoffrey Burnstock Prof Kate Bushby Mr Timothy Byrne Fr Brendan Callaghan

Dr Sheila Callender Sir Kenneth Calman Prof Hilary Calvert Prof Dugald Cameron

Prof Stewart Cameron Prof Alastair Campbell Dr Ian Campbell Prof Peter Campbell

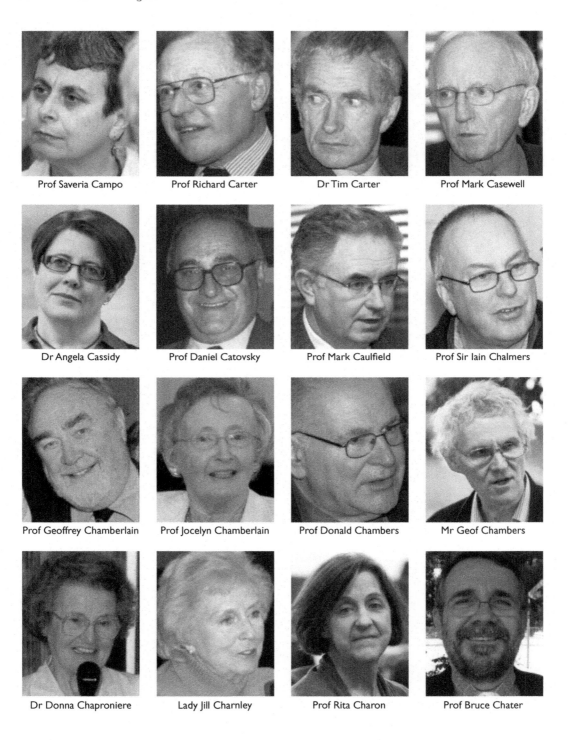

Prof Saveria Campo

Prof Richard Carter

Dr Tim Carter

Prof Mark Casewell

Dr Angela Cassidy

Prof Daniel Catovsky

Prof Mark Caulfield

Prof Sir Iain Chalmers

Prof Geoffrey Chamberlain

Prof Jocelyn Chamberlain

Prof Donald Chambers

Mr Geof Chambers

Dr Donna Chaproniere

Lady Jill Charnley

Prof Rita Charon

Prof Bruce Chater

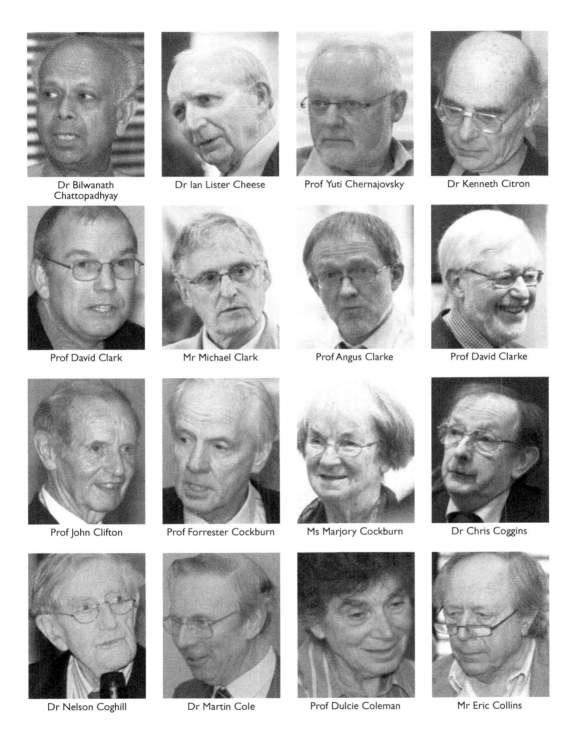

Dr Bilwanath
Chattopadhyay

Dr Ian Lister Cheese

Prof Yuti Chernajovsky

Dr Kenneth Citron

Prof David Clark

Mr Michael Clark

Prof Angus Clarke

Prof David Clarke

Prof John Clifton

Prof Forrester Cockburn

Ms Marjory Cockburn

Dr Chris Coggins

Dr Nelson Coghill

Dr Martin Cole

Prof Dulcie Coleman

Mr Eric Collins

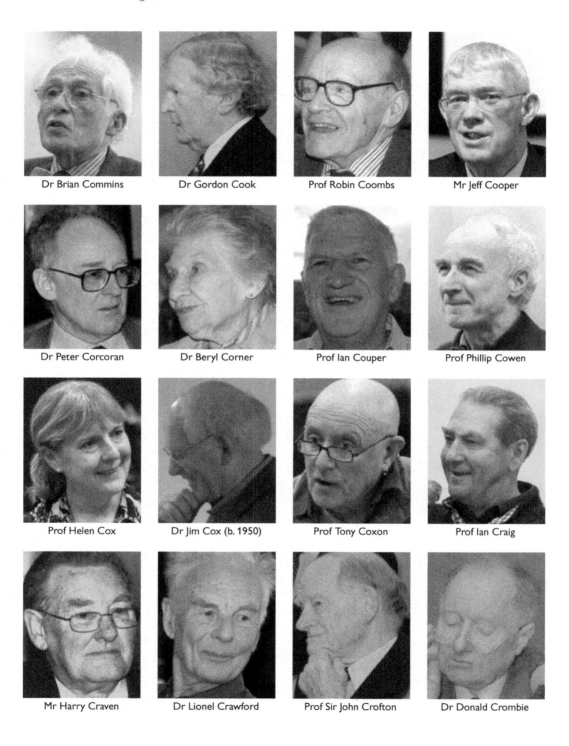

Dr Brian Commins

Dr Gordon Cook

Prof Robin Coombs

Mr Jeff Cooper

Dr Peter Corcoran

Dr Beryl Corner

Prof Ian Couper

Prof Phillip Cowen

Prof Helen Cox

Dr Jim Cox (b. 1950)

Prof Tony Coxon

Prof Ian Craig

Mr Harry Craven

Dr Lionel Crawford

Prof Sir John Crofton

Dr Donald Crombie

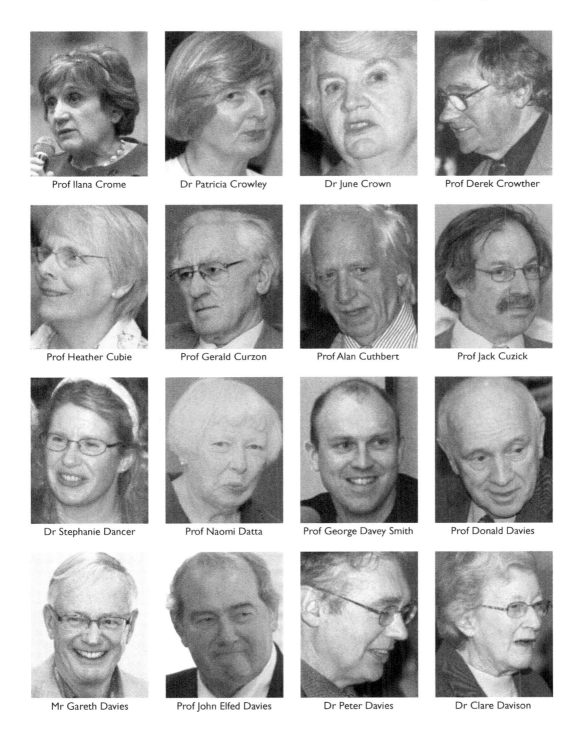

Prof Ilana Crome   Dr Patricia Crowley   Dr June Crown   Prof Derek Crowther

Prof Heather Cubie   Prof Gerald Curzon   Prof Alan Cuthbert   Prof Jack Cuzick

Dr Stephanie Dancer   Prof Naomi Datta   Prof George Davey Smith   Prof Donald Davies

Mr Gareth Davies   Prof John Elfed Davies   Dr Peter Davies   Dr Clare Davison

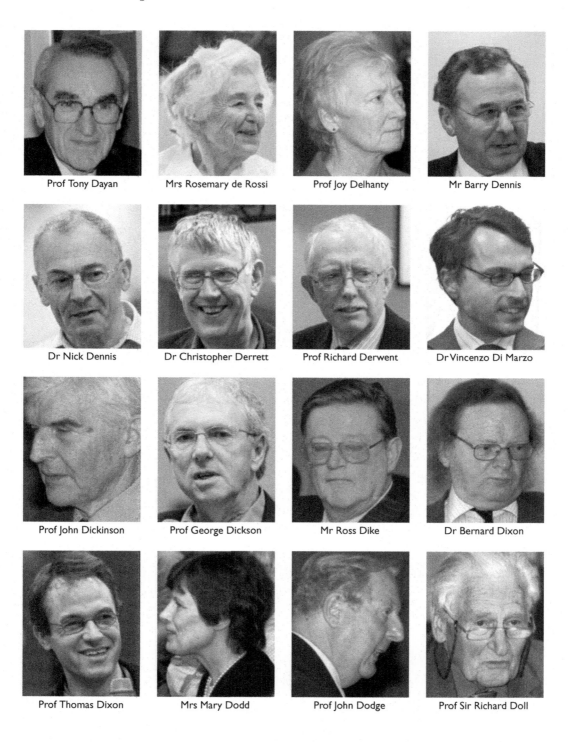

Prof Tony Dayan

Mrs Rosemary de Rossi

Prof Joy Delhanty

Mr Barry Dennis

Dr Nick Dennis

Dr Christopher Derrett

Prof Richard Derwent

Dr Vincenzo Di Marzo

Prof John Dickinson

Prof George Dickson

Mr Ross Dike

Dr Bernard Dixon

Prof Thomas Dixon

Mrs Mary Dodd

Prof John Dodge

Prof Sir Richard Doll

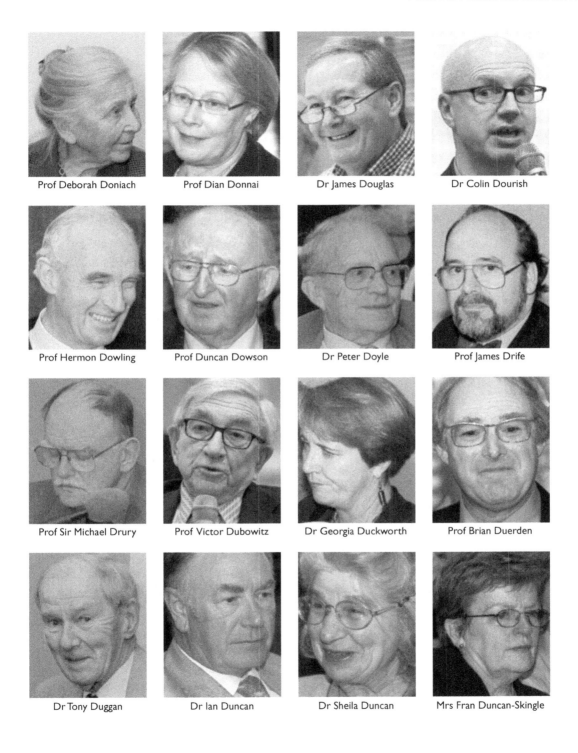

Prof Deborah Doniach

Prof Dian Donnai

Dr James Douglas

Dr Colin Dourish

Prof Hermon Dowling

Prof Duncan Dowson

Dr Peter Doyle

Prof James Drife

Prof Sir Michael Drury

Prof Victor Dubowitz

Dr Georgia Duckworth

Prof Brian Duerden

Dr Tony Duggan

Dr Ian Duncan

Dr Sheila Duncan

Mrs Fran Duncan-Skingle

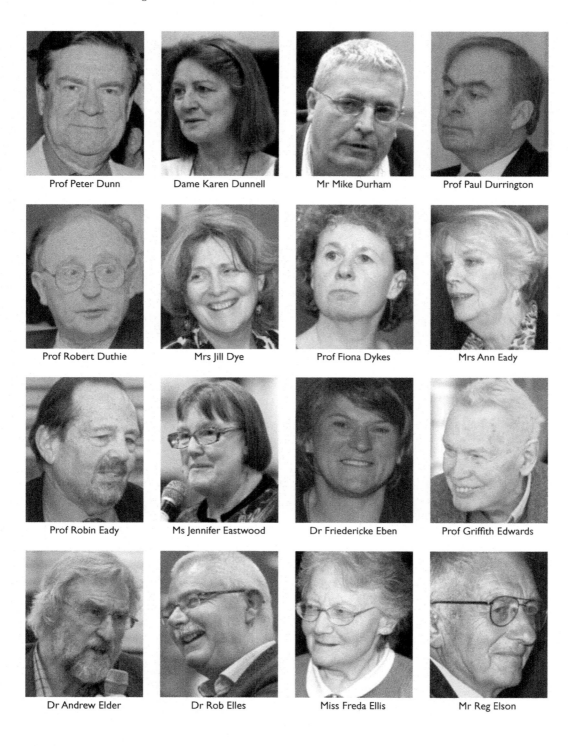

Prof Peter Dunn   Dame Karen Dunnell   Mr Mike Durham   Prof Paul Durrington

Prof Robert Duthie   Mrs Jill Dye   Prof Fiona Dykes   Mrs Ann Eady

Prof Robin Eady   Ms Jennifer Eastwood   Dr Friedericke Eben   Prof Griffith Edwards

Dr Andrew Elder   Dr Rob Elles   Miss Freda Ellis   Mr Reg Elson

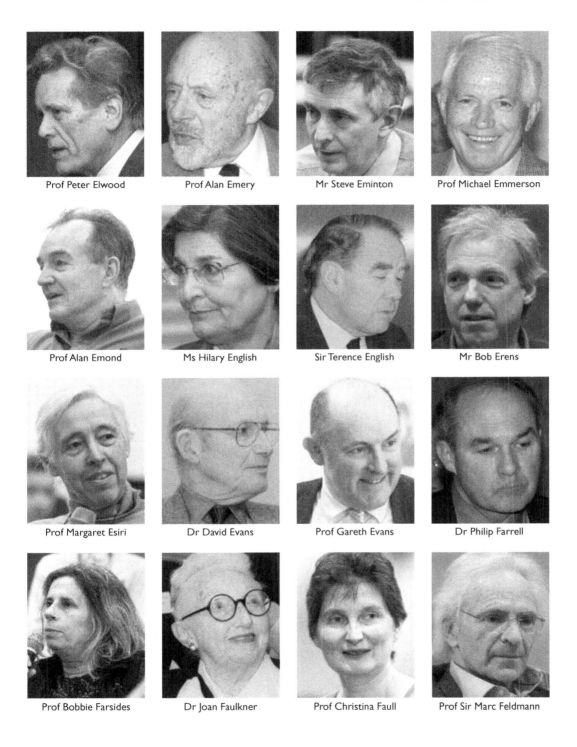

Prof Peter Elwood Prof Alan Emery Mr Steve Eminton Prof Michael Emmerson

Prof Alan Emond Ms Hilary English Sir Terence English Mr Bob Erens

Prof Margaret Esiri Dr David Evans Prof Gareth Evans Dr Philip Farrell

Prof Bobbie Farsides Dr Joan Faulkner Prof Christina Faull Prof Sir Marc Feldmann

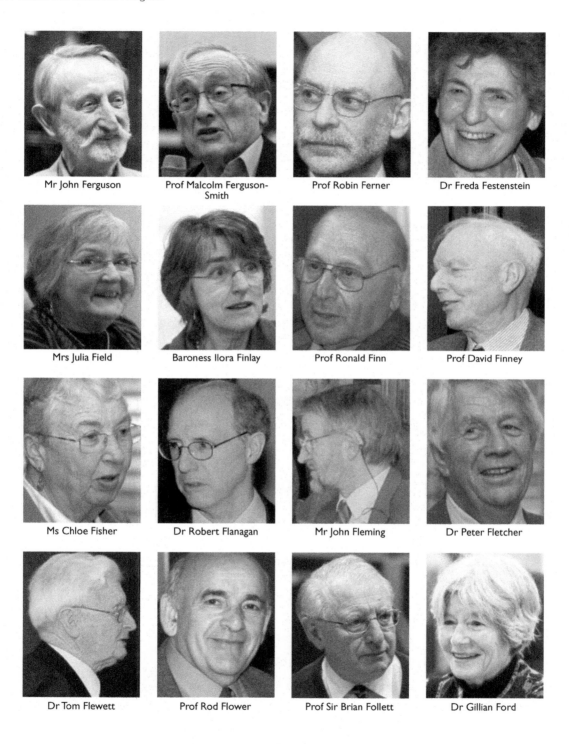

Mr John Ferguson

Prof Malcolm Ferguson-Smith

Prof Robin Ferner

Dr Freda Festenstein

Mrs Julia Field

Baroness Ilora Finlay

Prof Ronald Finn

Prof David Finney

Ms Chloe Fisher

Dr Robert Flanagan

Mr John Fleming

Dr Peter Fletcher

Dr Tom Flewett

Prof Rod Flower

Prof Sir Brian Follett

Dr Gillian Ford

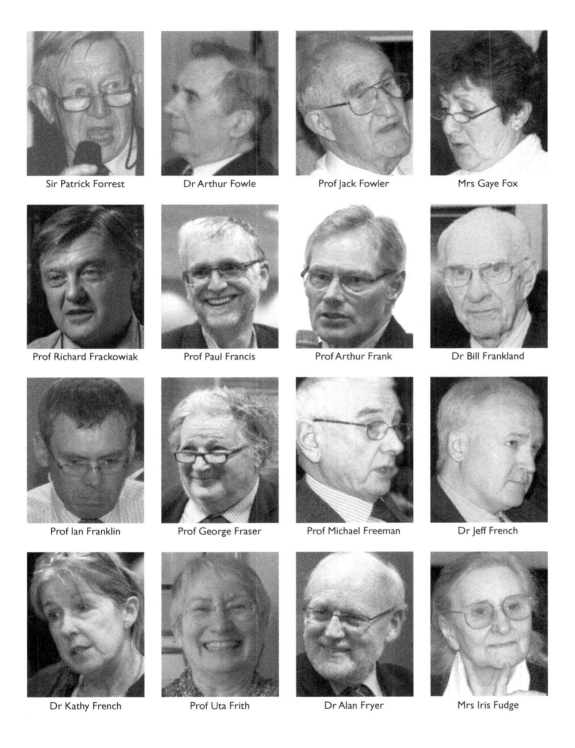

Sir Patrick Forrest

Dr Arthur Fowle

Prof Jack Fowler

Mrs Gaye Fox

Prof Richard Frackowiak

Prof Paul Francis

Prof Arthur Frank

Dr Bill Frankland

Prof Ian Franklin

Prof George Fraser

Prof Michael Freeman

Dr Jeff French

Dr Kathy French

Prof Uta Frith

Dr Alan Fryer

Mrs Iris Fudge

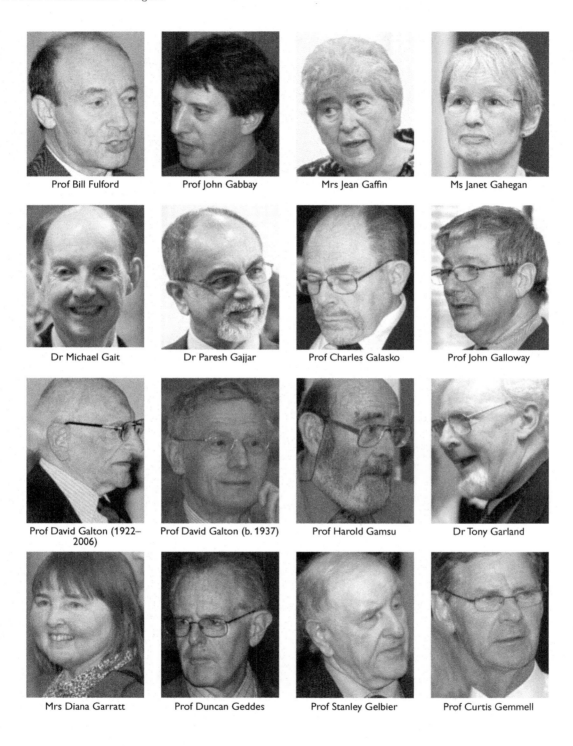

Prof Bill Fulford

Prof John Gabbay

Mrs Jean Gaffin

Ms Janet Gahegan

Dr Michael Gait

Dr Paresh Gajjar

Prof Charles Galasko

Prof John Galloway

Prof David Galton (1922–2006)

Prof David Galton (b. 1937)

Prof Harold Gamsu

Dr Tony Garland

Mrs Diana Garratt

Prof Duncan Geddes

Prof Stanley Gelbier

Prof Curtis Gemmell

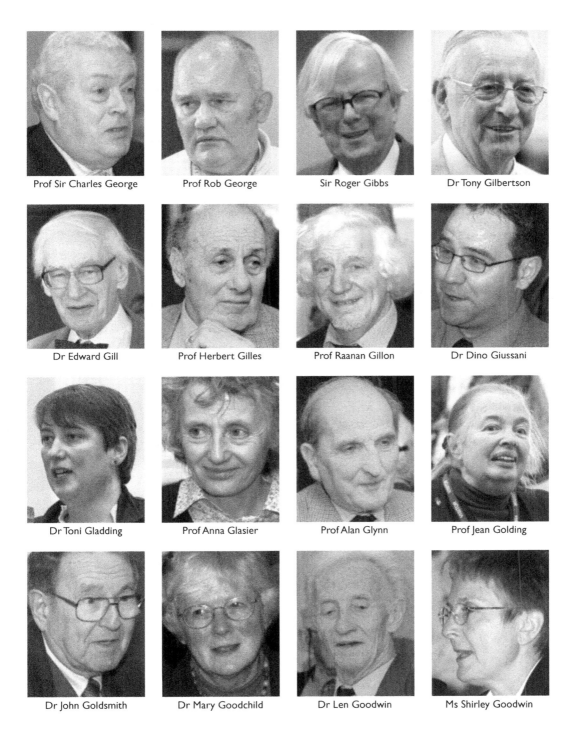

Prof Sir Charles George   Prof Rob George   Sir Roger Gibbs   Dr Tony Gilbertson

Dr Edward Gill   Prof Herbert Gilles   Prof Raanan Gillon   Dr Dino Giussani

Dr Toni Gladding   Prof Anna Glasier   Prof Alan Glynn   Prof Jean Golding

Dr John Goldsmith   Dr Mary Goodchild   Dr Len Goodwin   Ms Shirley Goodwin

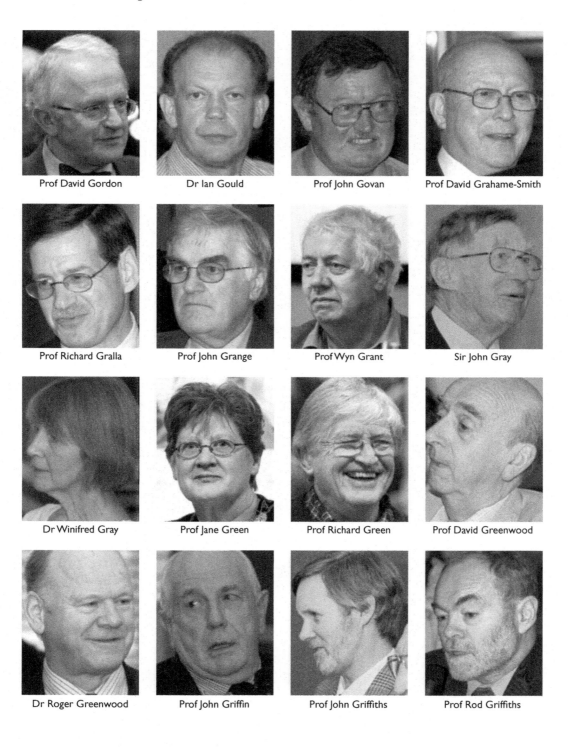

Prof David Gordon   Dr Ian Gould   Prof John Govan   Prof David Grahame-Smith

Prof Richard Gralla   Prof John Grange   Prof Wyn Grant   Sir John Gray

Dr Winifred Gray   Prof Jane Green   Prof Richard Green   Prof David Greenwood

Dr Roger Greenwood   Prof John Griffin   Prof John Griffiths   Prof Rod Griffiths

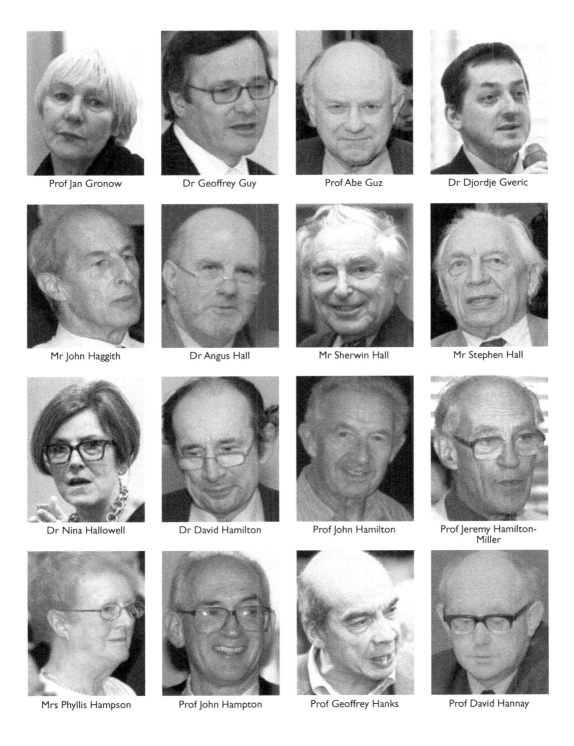

Prof Jan Gronow

Dr Geoffrey Guy

Prof Abe Guz

Dr Djordje Gveric

Mr John Haggith

Dr Angus Hall

Mr Sherwin Hall

Mr Stephen Hall

Dr Nina Hallowell

Dr David Hamilton

Prof John Hamilton

Prof Jeremy Hamilton-Miller

Mrs Phyllis Hampson

Prof John Hampton

Prof Geoffrey Hanks

Prof David Hannay

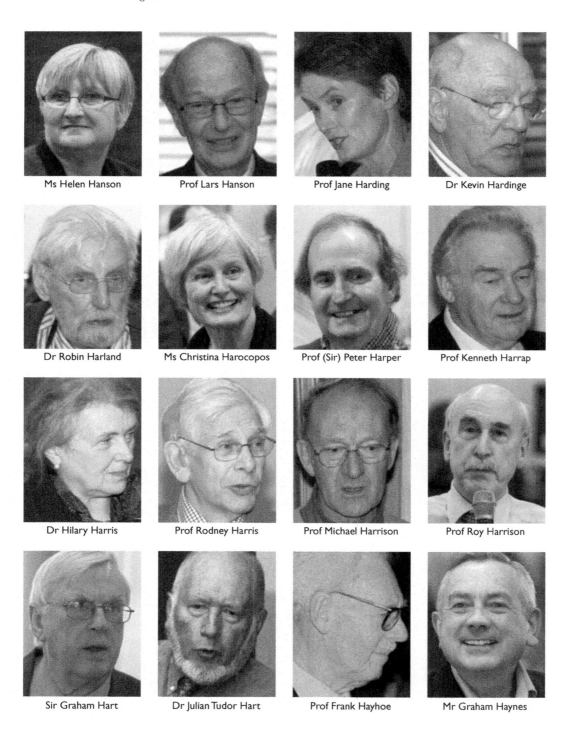

Ms Helen Hanson

Prof Lars Hanson

Prof Jane Harding

Dr Kevin Hardinge

Dr Robin Harland

Ms Christina Harocopos

Prof (Sir) Peter Harper

Prof Kenneth Harrap

Dr Hilary Harris

Prof Rodney Harris

Prof Michael Harrison

Prof Roy Harrison

Sir Graham Hart

Dr Julian Tudor Hart

Prof Frank Hayhoe

Mr Graham Haynes

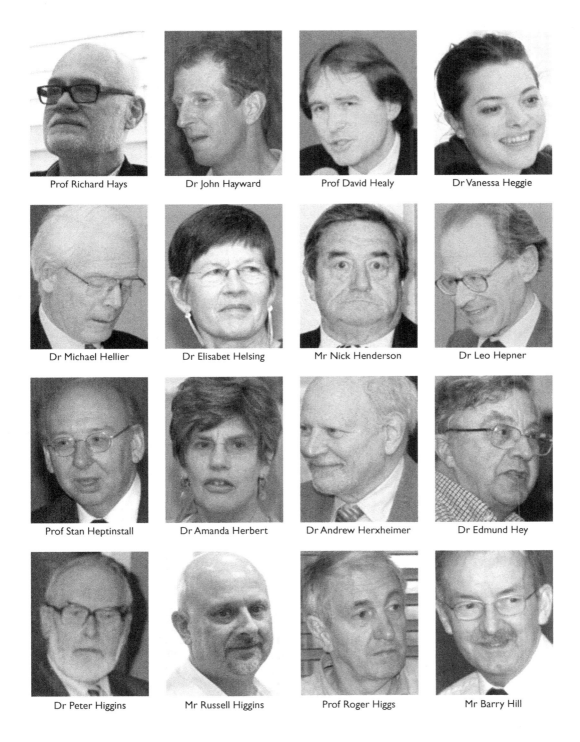

Prof Richard Hays Dr John Hayward Prof David Healy Dr Vanessa Heggie

Dr Michael Hellier Dr Elisabet Helsing Mr Nick Henderson Dr Leo Hepner

Prof Stan Heptinstall Dr Amanda Herbert Dr Andrew Herxheimer Dr Edmund Hey

Dr Peter Higgins Mr Russell Higgins Prof Roger Higgs Mr Barry Hill

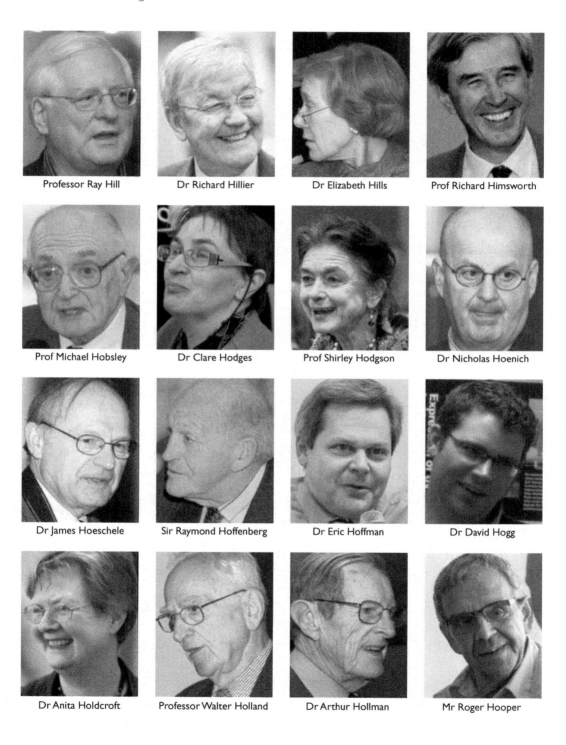

Professor Ray Hill

Dr Richard Hillier

Dr Elizabeth Hills

Prof Richard Himsworth

Prof Michael Hobsley

Dr Clare Hodges

Prof Shirley Hodgson

Dr Nicholas Hoenich

Dr James Hoeschele

Sir Raymond Hoffenberg

Dr Eric Hoffman

Dr David Hogg

Dr Anita Holdcroft

Professor Walter Holland

Dr Arthur Hollman

Mr Roger Hooper

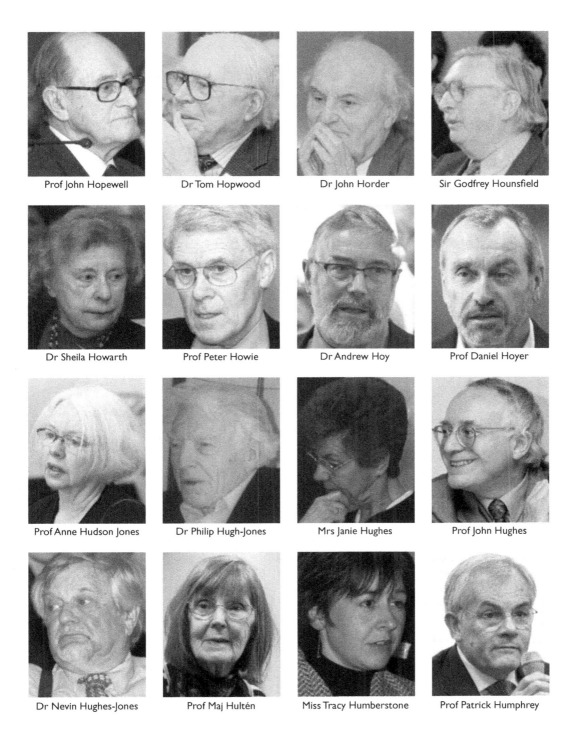

Prof John Hopewell Dr Tom Hopwood Dr John Horder Sir Godfrey Hounsfield

Dr Sheila Howarth Prof Peter Howie Dr Andrew Hoy Prof Daniel Hoyer

Prof Anne Hudson Jones Dr Philip Hugh-Jones Mrs Janie Hughes Prof John Hughes

Dr Nevin Hughes-Jones Prof Maj Hultén Miss Tracy Humberstone Prof Patrick Humphrey

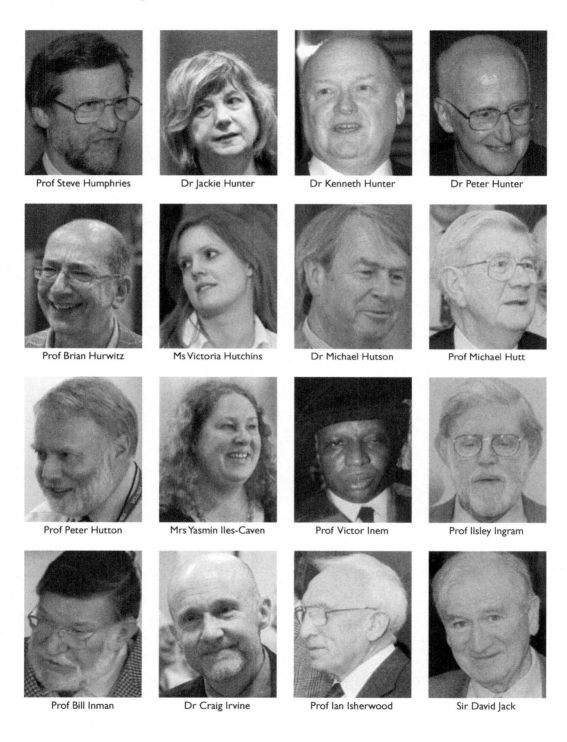

Prof Steve Humphries

Dr Jackie Hunter

Dr Kenneth Hunter

Dr Peter Hunter

Prof Brian Hurwitz

Ms Victoria Hutchins

Dr Michael Hutson

Prof Michael Hutt

Prof Peter Hutton

Mrs Yasmin Iles-Caven

Prof Victor Inem

Prof Ilsley Ingram

Prof Bill Inman

Dr Craig Irvine

Prof Ian Isherwood

Sir David Jack

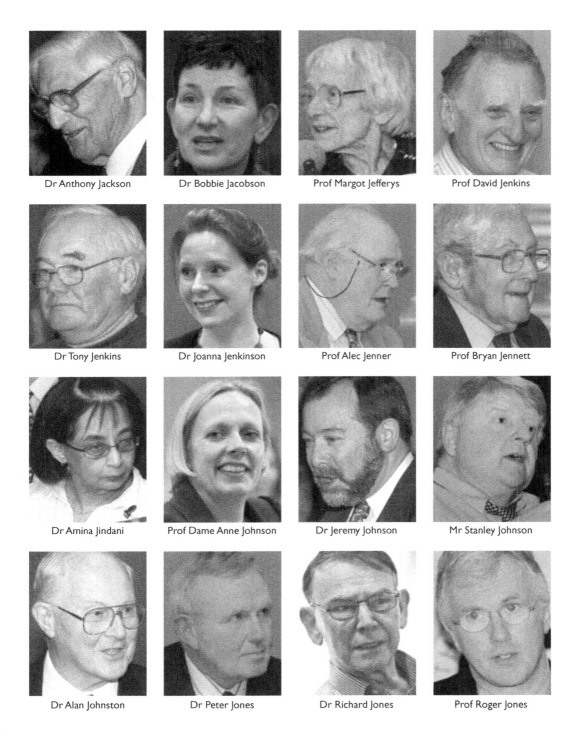

Dr Anthony Jackson   Dr Bobbie Jacobson   Prof Margot Jefferys   Prof David Jenkins

Dr Tony Jenkins   Dr Joanna Jenkinson   Prof Alec Jenner   Prof Bryan Jennett

Dr Amina Jindani   Prof Dame Anne Johnson   Dr Jeremy Johnson   Mr Stanley Johnson

Dr Alan Johnston   Dr Peter Jones   Dr Richard Jones   Prof Roger Jones

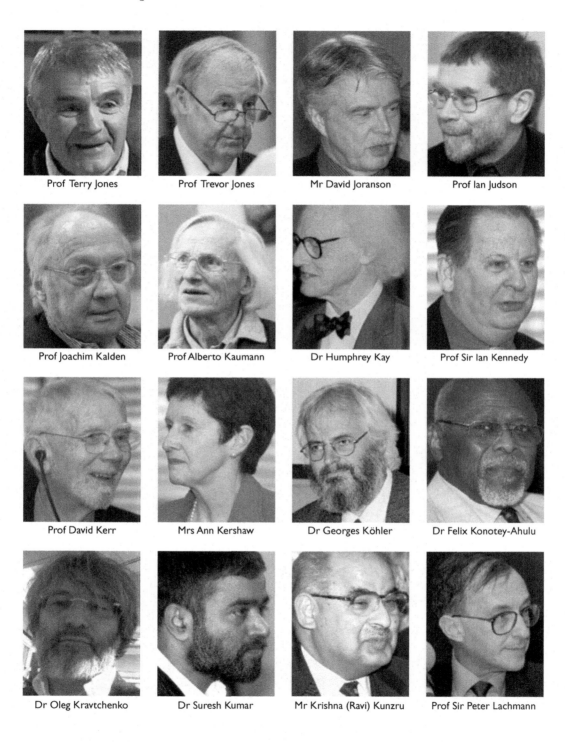

Prof Terry Jones

Prof Trevor Jones

Mr David Joranson

Prof Ian Judson

Prof Joachim Kalden

Prof Alberto Kaumann

Dr Humphrey Kay

Prof Sir Ian Kennedy

Prof David Kerr

Mrs Ann Kershaw

Dr Georges Köhler

Dr Felix Konotey-Ahulu

Dr Oleg Kravtchenko

Dr Suresh Kumar

Mr Krishna (Ravi) Kunzru

Prof Sir Peter Lachmann

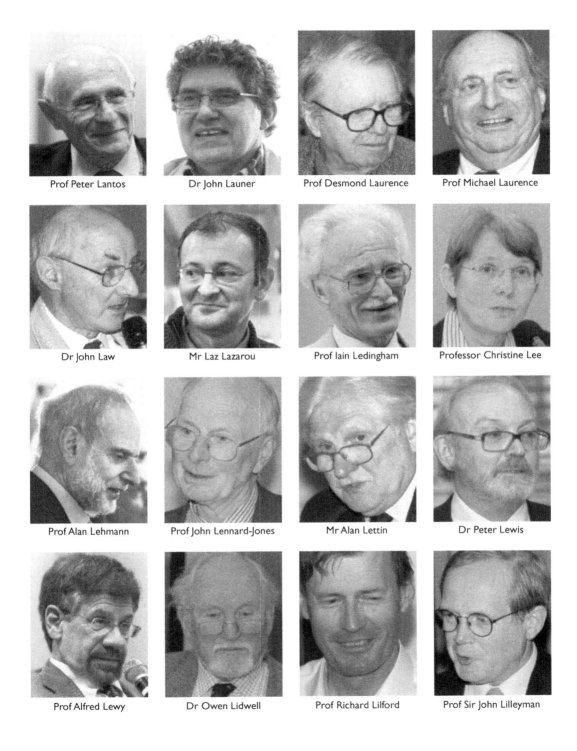

Prof Peter Lantos

Dr John Launer

Prof Desmond Laurence

Prof Michael Laurence

Dr John Law

Mr Laz Lazarou

Prof Iain Ledingham

Professor Christine Lee

Prof Alan Lehmann

Prof John Lennard-Jones

Mr Alan Lettin

Dr Peter Lewis

Prof Alfred Lewy

Dr Owen Lidwell

Prof Richard Lilford

Prof Sir John Lilleyman

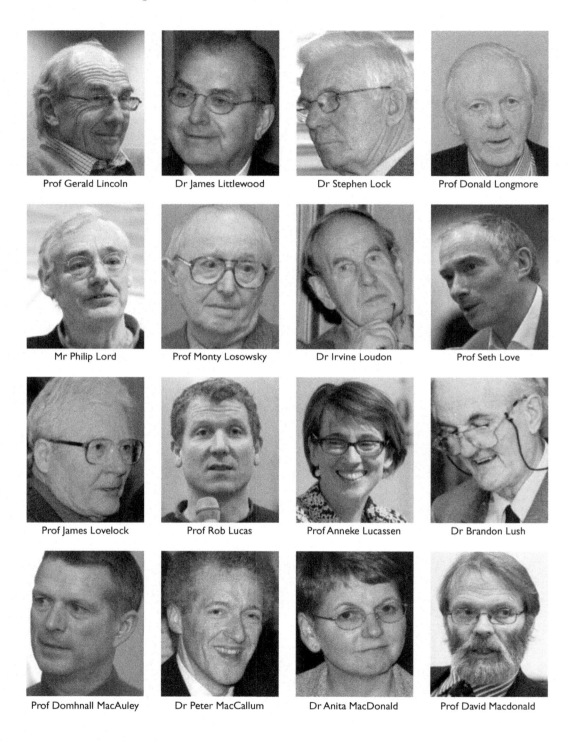

Prof Gerald Lincoln

Dr James Littlewood

Dr Stephen Lock

Prof Donald Longmore

Mr Philip Lord

Prof Monty Losowsky

Dr Irvine Loudon

Prof Seth Love

Prof James Lovelock

Prof Rob Lucas

Prof Anneke Lucassen

Dr Brandon Lush

Prof Domhnall MacAuley

Dr Peter MacCallum

Dr Anita MacDonald

Prof David Macdonald

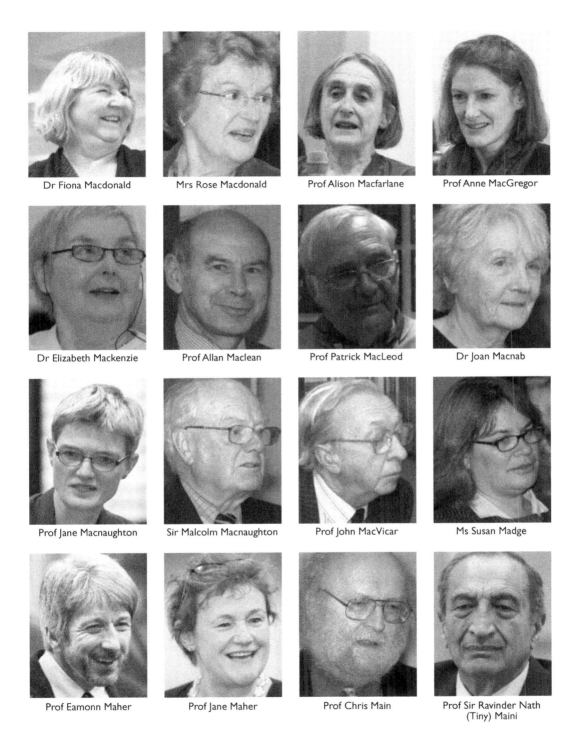

Dr Fiona Macdonald

Mrs Rose Macdonald

Prof Alison Macfarlane

Prof Anne MacGregor

Dr Elizabeth Mackenzie

Prof Allan Maclean

Prof Patrick MacLeod

Dr Joan Macnab

Prof Jane Macnaughton

Sir Malcolm Macnaughton

Prof John MacVicar

Ms Susan Madge

Prof Eamonn Maher

Prof Jane Maher

Prof Chris Main

Prof Sir Ravinder Nath
(Tiny) Maini

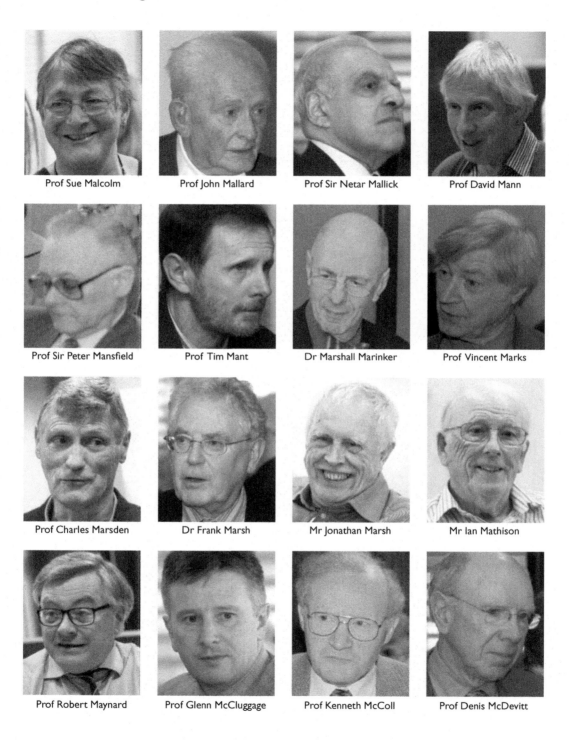

Prof Sue Malcolm   Prof John Mallard   Prof Sir Netar Mallick   Prof David Mann

Prof Sir Peter Mansfield   Prof Tim Mant   Dr Marshall Marinker   Prof Vincent Marks

Prof Charles Marsden   Dr Frank Marsh   Mr Jonathan Marsh   Mr Ian Mathison

Prof Robert Maynard   Prof Glenn McCluggage   Prof Kenneth McColl   Prof Denis McDevitt

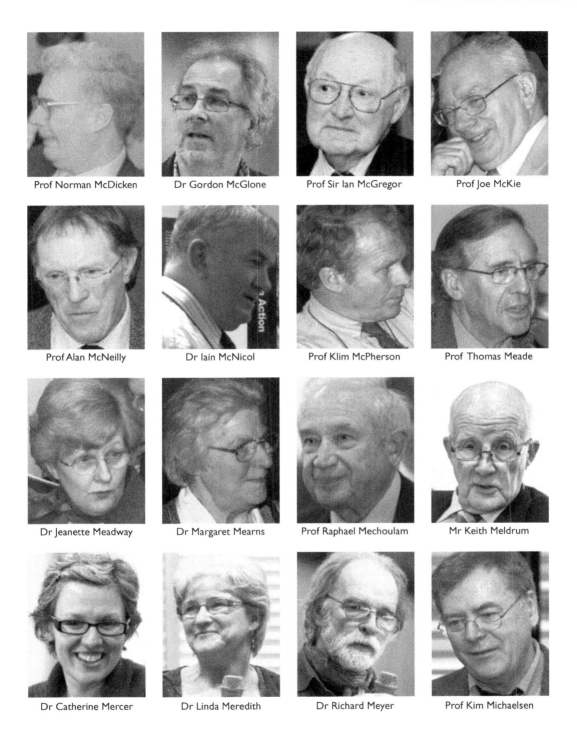

Prof Norman McDicken   Dr Gordon McGlone   Prof Sir Ian McGregor   Prof Joe McKie

Prof Alan McNeilly   Dr Iain McNicol   Prof Klim McPherson   Prof Thomas Meade

Dr Jeanette Meadway   Dr Margaret Mearns   Prof Raphael Mechoulam   Mr Keith Meldrum

Dr Catherine Mercer   Dr Linda Meredith   Dr Richard Meyer   Prof Kim Michaelsen

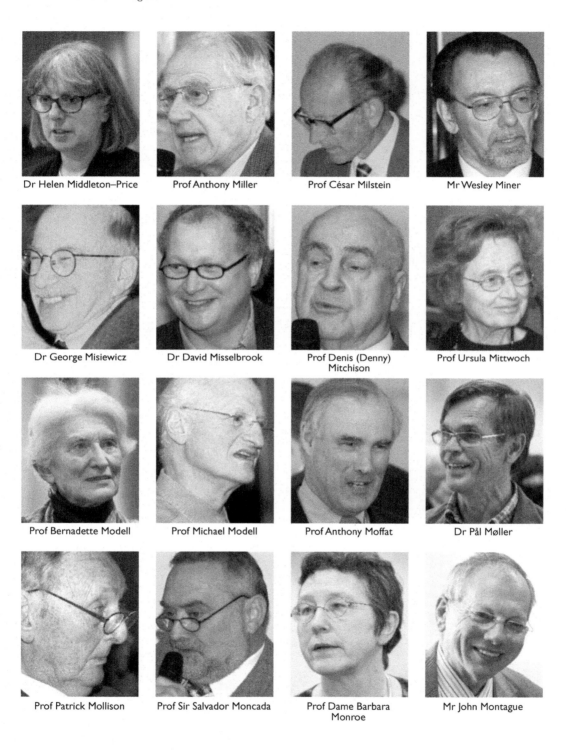

Dr Helen Middleton–Price

Prof Anthony Miller

Prof César Milstein

Mr Wesley Miner

Dr George Misiewicz

Dr David Misselbrook

Prof Denis (Denny) Mitchison

Prof Ursula Mittwoch

Prof Bernadette Modell

Prof Michael Modell

Prof Anthony Moffat

Dr Pål Møller

Prof Patrick Mollison

Prof Sir Salvador Moncada

Prof Dame Barbara Monroe

Mr John Montague

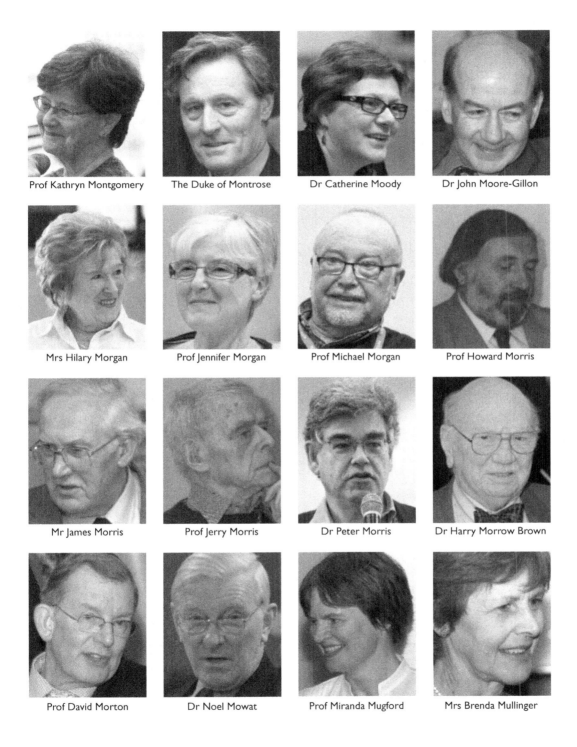

Prof Kathryn Montgomery	The Duke of Montrose	Dr Catherine Moody	Dr John Moore-Gillon
Mrs Hilary Morgan	Prof Jennifer Morgan	Prof Michael Morgan	Prof Howard Morris
Mr James Morris	Prof Jerry Morris	Dr Peter Morris	Dr Harry Morrow Brown
Prof David Morton	Dr Noel Mowat	Prof Miranda Mugford	Mrs Brenda Mullinger

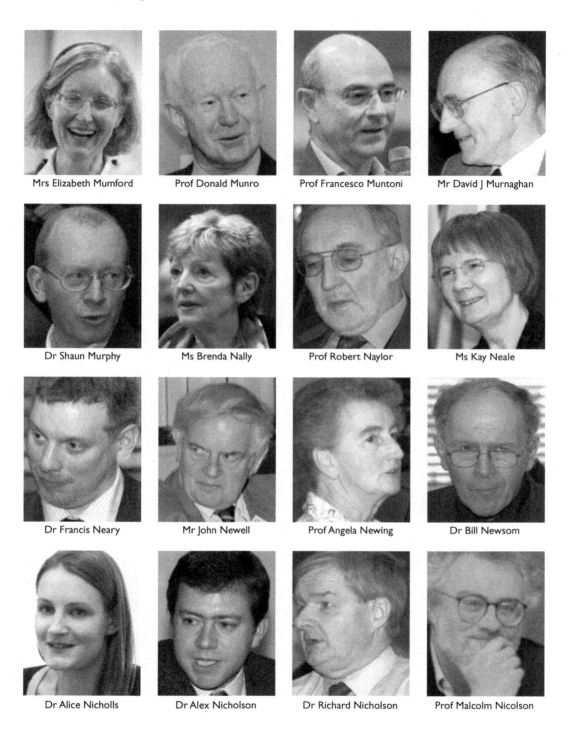

Mrs Elizabeth Mumford

Prof Donald Munro

Prof Francesco Muntoni

Mr David J Murnaghan

Dr Shaun Murphy

Ms Brenda Nally

Prof Robert Naylor

Ms Kay Neale

Dr Francis Neary

Mr John Newell

Prof Angela Newing

Dr Bill Newsom

Dr Alice Nicholls

Dr Alex Nicholson

Dr Richard Nicholson

Prof Malcolm Nicolson

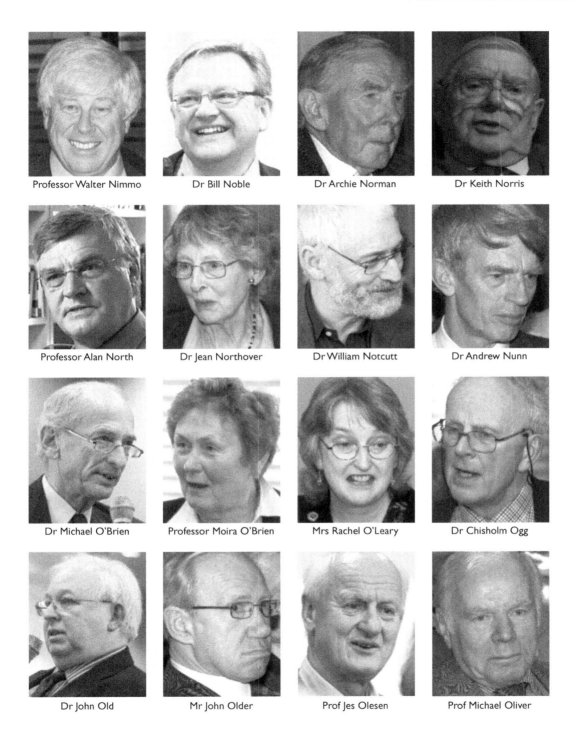

Professor Walter Nimmo

Dr Bill Noble

Dr Archie Norman

Dr Keith Norris

Professor Alan North

Dr Jean Northover

Dr William Notcutt

Dr Andrew Nunn

Dr Michael O'Brien

Professor Moira O'Brien

Mrs Rachel O'Leary

Dr Chisholm Ogg

Dr John Old

Mr John Older

Prof Jes Olesen

Prof Michael Oliver

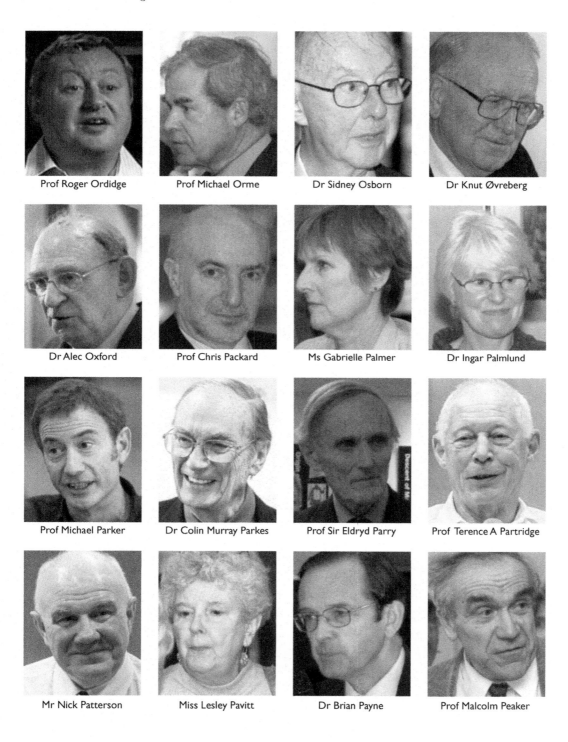

Prof Roger Ordidge   Prof Michael Orme   Dr Sidney Osborn   Dr Knut Øvreberg

Dr Alec Oxford   Prof Chris Packard   Ms Gabrielle Palmer   Dr Ingar Palmlund

Prof Michael Parker   Dr Colin Murray Parkes   Prof Sir Eldryd Parry   Prof Terence A Partridge

Mr Nick Patterson   Miss Lesley Pavitt   Dr Brian Payne   Prof Malcolm Peaker

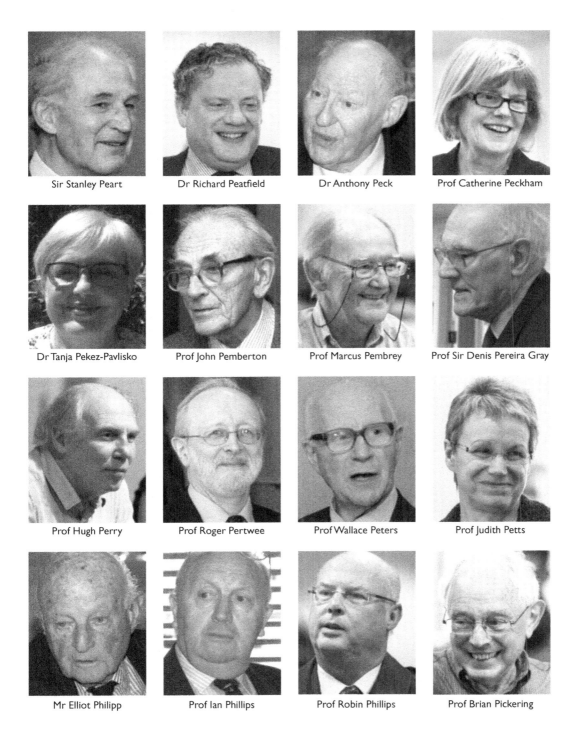

Sir Stanley Peart | Dr Richard Peatfield | Dr Anthony Peck | Prof Catherine Peckham

Dr Tanja Pekez-Pavlisko | Prof John Pemberton | Prof Marcus Pembrey | Prof Sir Denis Pereira Gray

Prof Hugh Perry | Prof Roger Pertwee | Prof Wallace Peters | Prof Judith Petts

Mr Elliot Philipp | Prof Ian Phillips | Prof Robin Phillips | Prof Brian Pickering

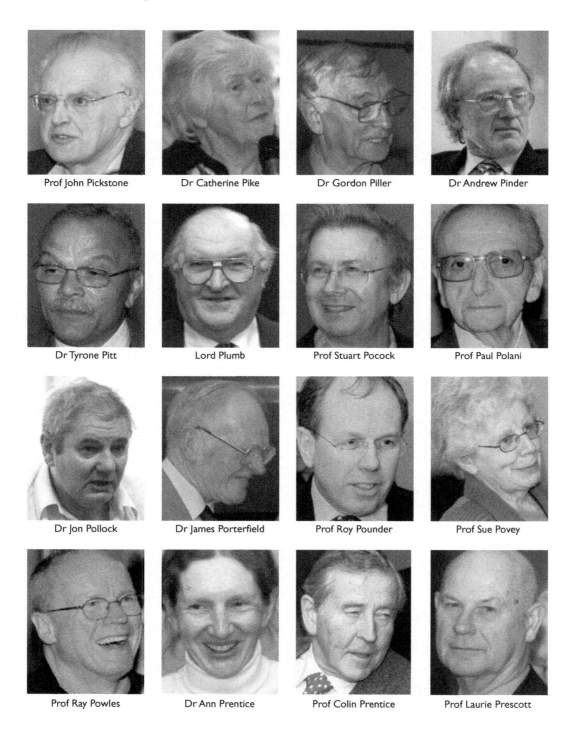

Prof John Pickstone

Dr Catherine Pike

Dr Gordon Piller

Dr Andrew Pinder

Dr Tyrone Pitt

Lord Plumb

Prof Stuart Pocock

Prof Paul Polani

Dr Jon Pollock

Dr James Porterfield

Prof Roy Pounder

Prof Sue Povey

Prof Ray Powles

Dr Ann Prentice

Prof Colin Prentice

Prof Laurie Prescott

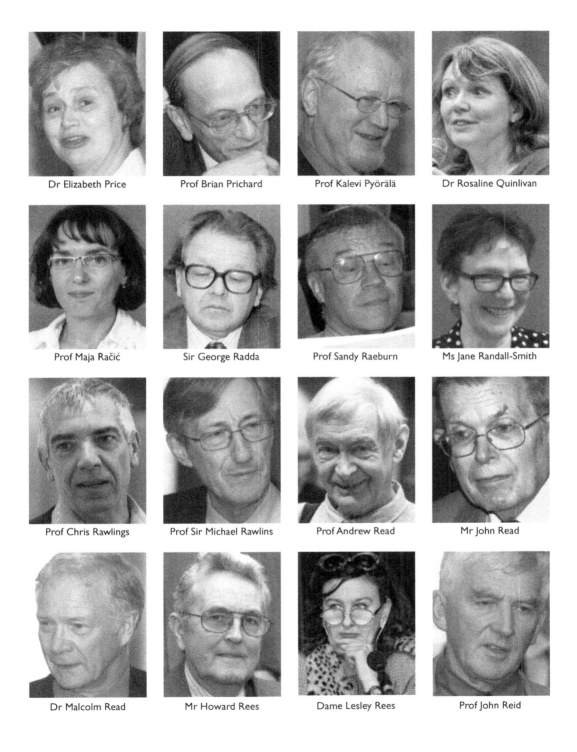

Dr Elizabeth Price

Prof Brian Prichard

Prof Kalevi Pyörälä

Dr Rosaline Quinlivan

Prof Maja Račić

Sir George Radda

Prof Sandy Raeburn

Ms Jane Randall-Smith

Prof Chris Rawlings

Prof Sir Michael Rawlins

Prof Andrew Read

Mr John Read

Dr Malcolm Read

Mr Howard Rees

Dame Lesley Rees

Prof John Reid

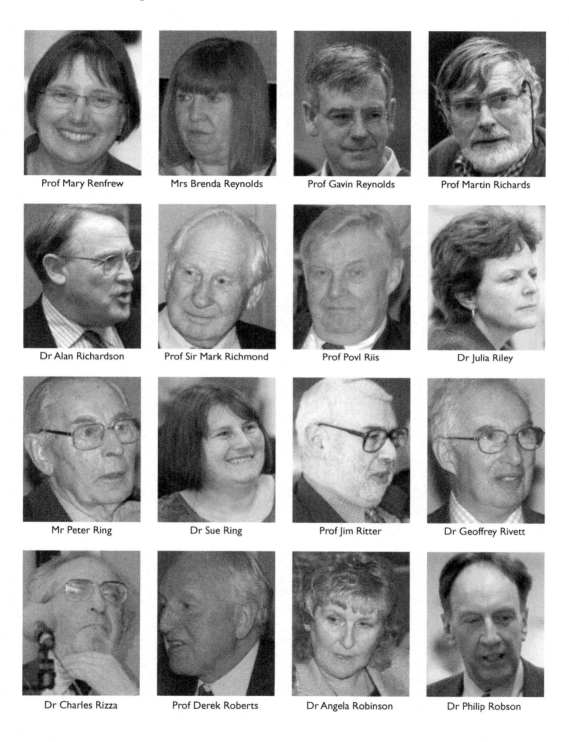

Prof Mary Renfrew

Mrs Brenda Reynolds

Prof Gavin Reynolds

Prof Martin Richards

Dr Alan Richardson

Prof Sir Mark Richmond

Prof Povl Riis

Dr Julia Riley

Mr Peter Ring

Dr Sue Ring

Prof Jim Ritter

Dr Geoffrey Rivett

Dr Charles Rizza

Prof Derek Roberts

Dr Angela Robinson

Dr Philip Robson

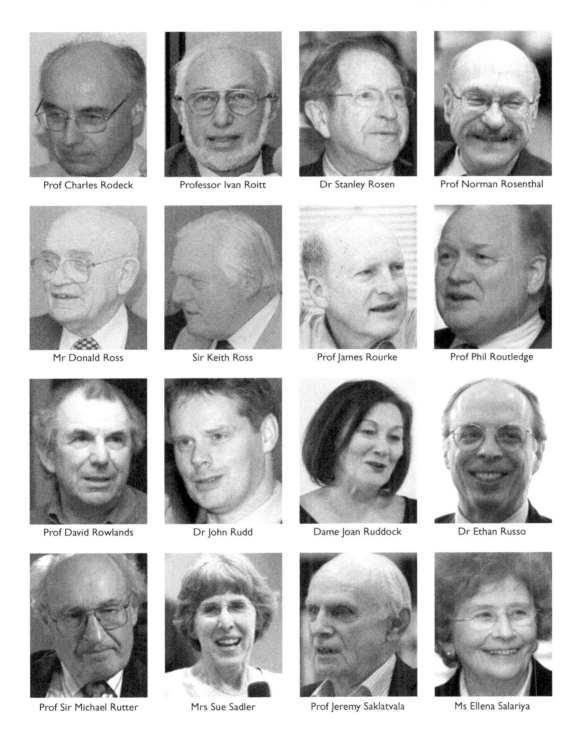

Prof Charles Rodeck

Professor Ivan Roitt

Dr Stanley Rosen

Prof Norman Rosenthal

Mr Donald Ross

Sir Keith Ross

Prof James Rourke

Prof Phil Routledge

Prof David Rowlands

Dr John Rudd

Dame Joan Ruddock

Dr Ethan Russo

Prof Sir Michael Rutter

Mrs Sue Sadler

Prof Jeremy Saklatvala

Ms Ellena Salariya

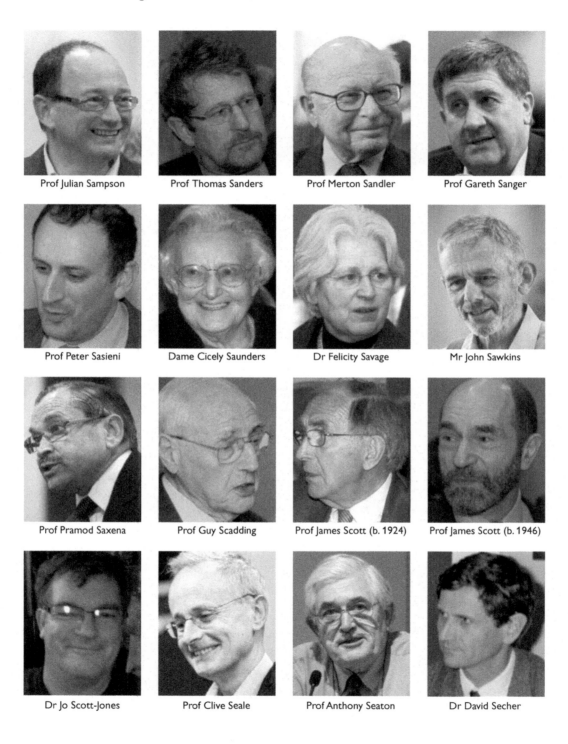

Prof Julian Sampson

Prof Thomas Sanders

Prof Merton Sandler

Prof Gareth Sanger

Prof Peter Sasieni

Dame Cicely Saunders

Dr Felicity Savage

Mr John Sawkins

Prof Pramod Saxena

Prof Guy Scadding

Prof James Scott (b. 1924)

Prof James Scott (b. 1946)

Dr Jo Scott-Jones

Prof Clive Seale

Prof Anthony Seaton

Dr David Secher

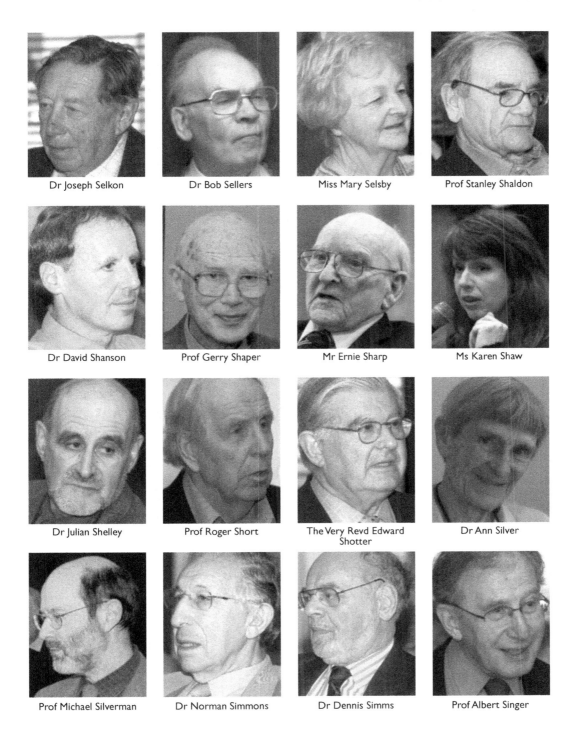

Dr Joseph Selkon

Dr Bob Sellers

Miss Mary Selsby

Prof Stanley Shaldon

Dr David Shanson

Prof Gerry Shaper

Mr Ernie Sharp

Ms Karen Shaw

Dr Julian Shelley

Prof Roger Short

The Very Revd Edward Shotter

Dr Ann Silver

Prof Michael Silverman

Dr Norman Simmons

Dr Dennis Simms

Prof Albert Singer

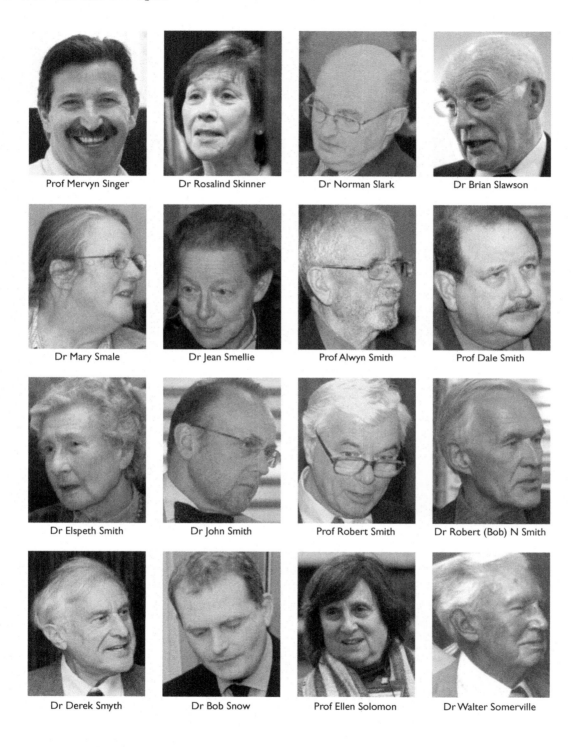

Prof Mervyn Singer   Dr Rosalind Skinner   Dr Norman Slark   Dr Brian Slawson

Dr Mary Smale   Dr Jean Smellie   Prof Alwyn Smith   Prof Dale Smith

Dr Elspeth Smith   Dr John Smith   Prof Robert Smith   Dr Robert (Bob) N Smith

Dr Derek Smyth   Dr Bob Snow   Prof Ellen Solomon   Dr Walter Somerville

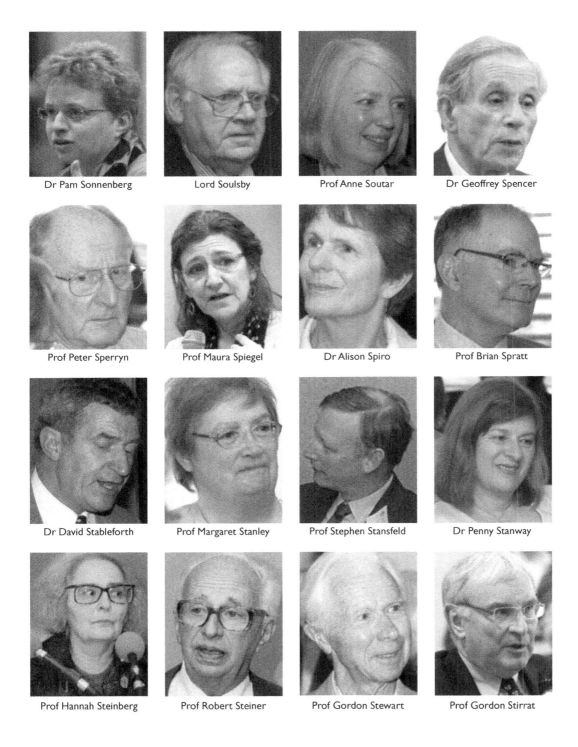

Dr Pam Sonnenberg

Lord Soulsby

Prof Anne Soutar

Dr Geoffrey Spencer

Prof Peter Sperryn

Prof Maura Spiegel

Dr Alison Spiro

Prof Brian Spratt

Dr David Stableforth

Prof Margaret Stanley

Prof Stephen Stansfeld

Dr Penny Stanway

Prof Hannah Steinberg

Prof Robert Steiner

Prof Gordon Stewart

Prof Gordon Stirrat

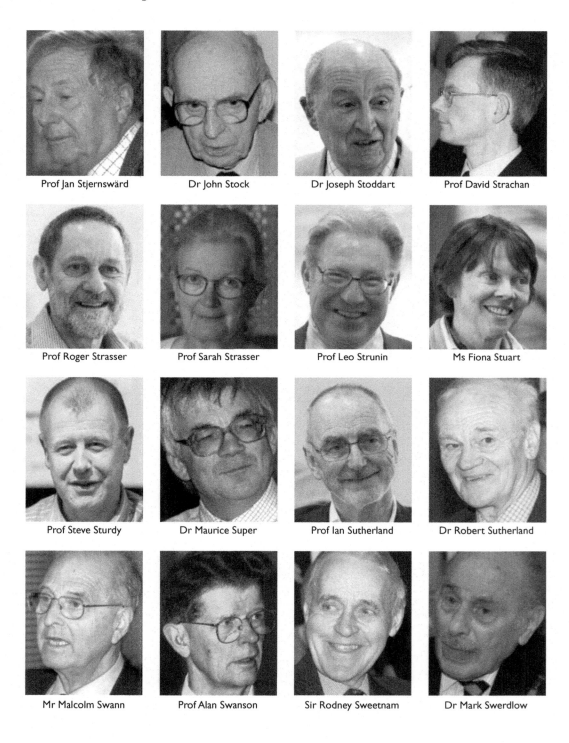

Prof Jan Stjernswärd

Dr John Stock

Dr Joseph Stoddart

Prof David Strachan

Prof Roger Strasser

Prof Sarah Strasser

Prof Leo Strunin

Ms Fiona Stuart

Prof Steve Sturdy

Dr Maurice Super

Prof Ian Sutherland

Dr Robert Sutherland

Mr Malcolm Swann

Prof Alan Swanson

Sir Rodney Sweetnam

Dr Mark Swerdlow

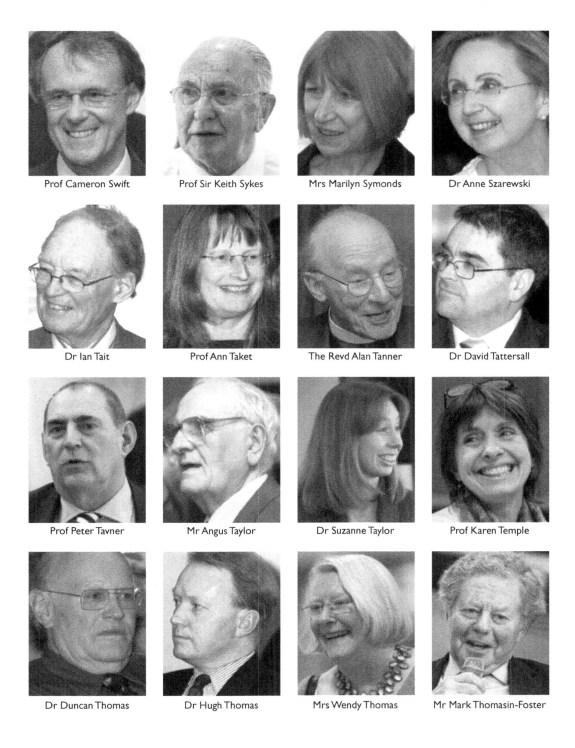

Prof Cameron Swift

Prof Sir Keith Sykes

Mrs Marilyn Symonds

Dr Anne Szarewski

Dr Ian Tait

Prof Ann Taket

The Revd Alan Tanner

Dr David Tattersall

Prof Peter Tavner

Mr Angus Taylor

Dr Suzanne Taylor

Prof Karen Temple

Dr Duncan Thomas

Dr Hugh Thomas

Mrs Wendy Thomas

Mr Mark Thomasin-Foster

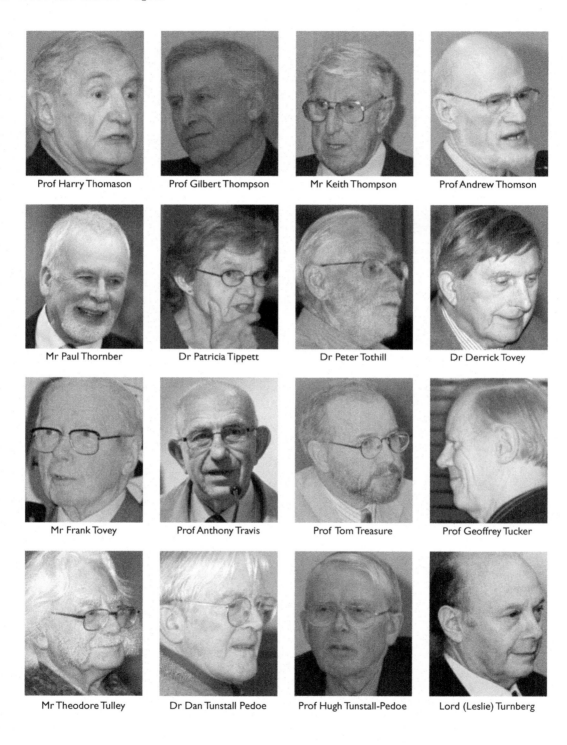

Prof Harry Thomason

Prof Gilbert Thompson

Mr Keith Thompson

Prof Andrew Thomson

Mr Paul Thornber

Dr Patricia Tippett

Dr Peter Tothill

Dr Derrick Tovey

Mr Frank Tovey

Prof Anthony Travis

Prof Tom Treasure

Prof Geoffrey Tucker

Mr Theodore Tulley

Dr Dan Tunstall Pedoe

Prof Hugh Tunstall-Pedoe

Lord (Leslie) Turnberg

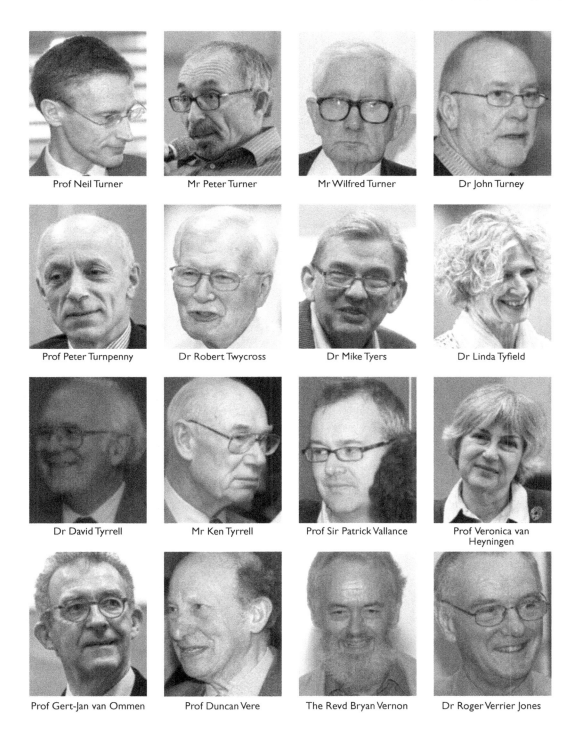

Prof Neil Turner

Mr Peter Turner

Mr Wilfred Turner

Dr John Turney

Prof Peter Turnpenny

Dr Robert Twycross

Dr Mike Tyers

Dr Linda Tyfield

Dr David Tyrrell

Mr Ken Tyrrell

Prof Sir Patrick Vallance

Prof Veronica van Heyningen

Prof Gert-Jan van Ommen

Prof Duncan Vere

The Revd Bryan Vernon

Dr Roger Verrier Jones

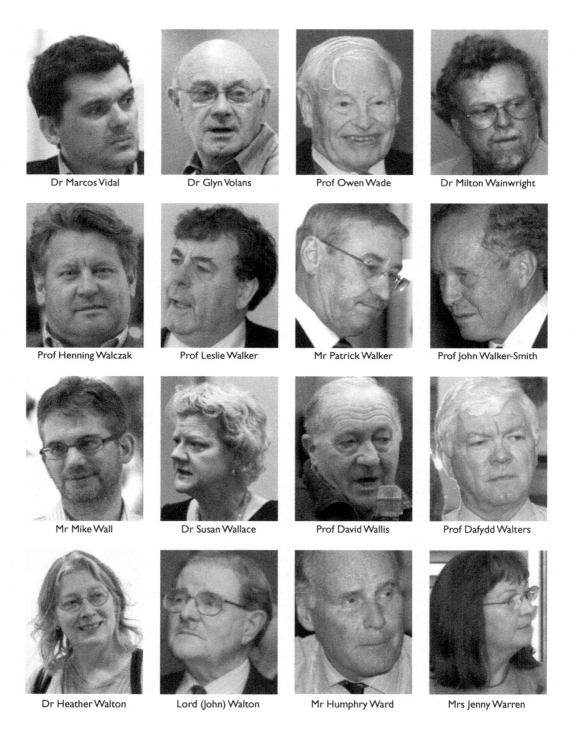

Dr Marcos Vidal   Dr Glyn Volans   Prof Owen Wade   Dr Milton Wainwright

Prof Henning Walczak   Prof Leslie Walker   Mr Patrick Walker   Prof John Walker-Smith

Mr Mike Wall   Dr Susan Wallace   Prof David Wallis   Prof Dafydd Walters

Dr Heather Walton   Lord (John) Walton   Mr Humphry Ward   Mrs Jenny Warren

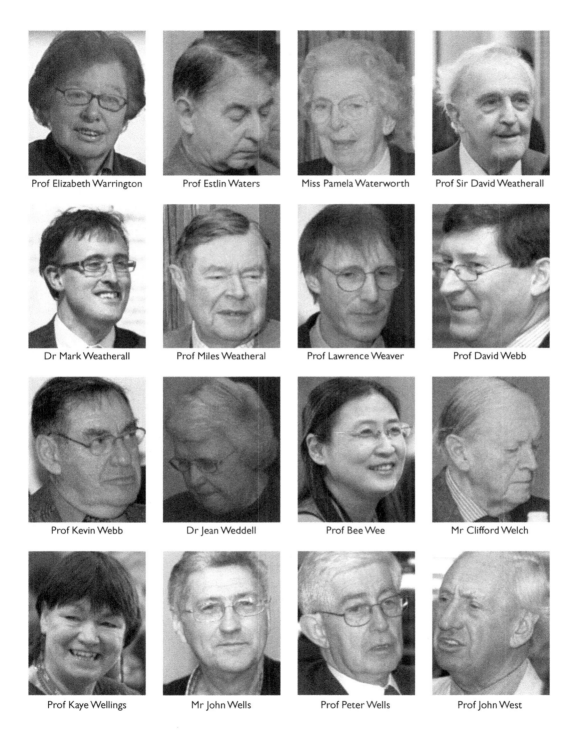

Prof Elizabeth Warrington

Prof Estlin Waters

Miss Pamela Waterworth

Prof Sir David Weatherall

Dr Mark Weatherall

Prof Miles Weatheral

Prof Lawrence Weaver

Prof David Webb

Prof Kevin Webb

Dr Jean Weddell

Prof Bee Wee

Mr Clifford Welch

Prof Kaye Wellings

Mr John Wells

Prof Peter Wells

Prof John West

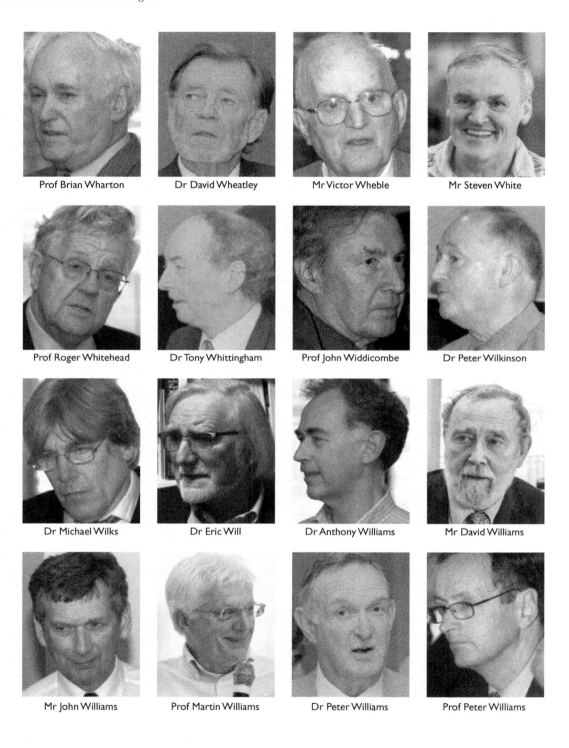

Prof Brian Wharton

Dr David Wheatley

Mr Victor Wheble

Mr Steven White

Prof Roger Whitehead

Dr Tony Whittingham

Prof John Widdicombe

Dr Peter Wilkinson

Dr Michael Wilks

Dr Eric Will

Dr Anthony Williams

Mr David Williams

Mr John Williams

Prof Martin Williams

Dr Peter Williams

Prof Peter Williams

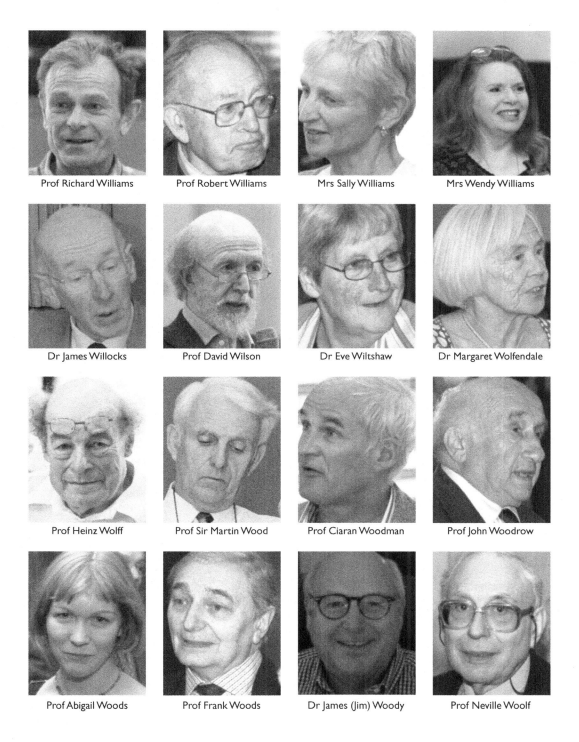

Prof Richard Williams   Prof Robert Williams   Mrs Sally Williams   Mrs Wendy Williams

Dr James Willocks   Prof David Wilson   Dr Eve Wiltshaw   Dr Margaret Wolfendale

Prof Heinz Wolff   Prof Sir Martin Wood   Prof Ciaran Woodman   Prof John Woodrow

Prof Abigail Woods   Prof Frank Woods   Dr James (Jim) Woody   Prof Neville Woolf

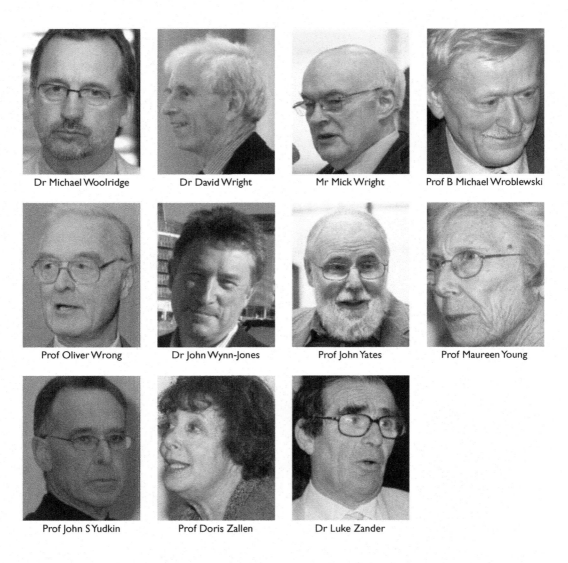

Dr Michael Woolridge

Dr David Wright

Mr Mick Wright

Prof B Michael Wroblewski

Prof Oliver Wrong

Dr John Wynn-Jones

Prof John Yates

Prof Maureen Young

Prof John S Yudkin

Prof Doris Zallen

Dr Luke Zander

Lightning Source UK Ltd.
Milton Keynes UK
UKOW04f0723210517
301562UK00001B/111/P